Cognitive Behaviour Therapy for People with Cancer

Cognitive behaviour therapy for people with cancer

by

Stirling Moorey, BSc, FRCPsych.
Consultant Psychiatrist in Cognitive Behaviour Therapy
Maudsley Hospital, London, UK

and

Steven Greer, MD, FRCPsych., FRANZCP
Consultant Psychiatrist
St Raphael's Hospice, North Cheam, Surrey, UK

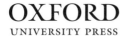

OXFORD
UNIVERSITY PRESS

OXFORD

UNIVERSITY PRESS

Great Clarendon Street, Oxford OX2 6DP

Oxford University Press is a department of the University of Oxford. It
furthers the University's objective of excellence in research, scholarship,
and education by publishing worldwide in

Oxford New York

Auckland Bangkok Buenos Aires Cape Town Chennai
Dar es Salaam Delhi Hong Kong Istanbul Karachi Kolkata
Kuala Lumpur Madrid Melbourne Mexico City Mumbai Nairobi
São Paulo Shanghai Taipei Tokyo Toronto

and an associated company in Berlin

Oxford is a registered trade mark of Oxford University Press in the UK
and in certain other countries

Published in the United States by Oxford University Press Inc., New York

First published under the title Psychological Therapy for Patients with
Cancer: A New Approach 1989 (Heinemann Medical Books)

This edition published 2002

A catalogue record for this title is available from the British Library

Library of Congress Cataloging in Publication Data
(Data available)

ISBN 0 19 850866 2 (Pbk)

10 9 8 7 6 5 4 3 2 1

Typeset by Cepha Imaging Pvt Ltd, India
Printed in Great Britain
on acid-free paper by Biddles Ltd, Guildford & King's Lynn

As no two persons are alike in health, so no two are alike in disease; and no diagnosis is complete or exact which does not include an estimate of the character or constitution of the patient ... for to treat a sick man rightly requires diagnosis not only of the disease but the manner and degrees in which its supposed essential characters are modified by his personal qualities, by the inheritances that converge in him, by the changes wrought in him by the conditions of his past life, and many things besides.

James Paget (1885)
Address to Abernethian Society

Foreword

This second edition of *Cognitive behaviour therapy for patients with cancer* underscores the significant role Stirling Moorey and Steven Greer play as leaders in the developing field of psycho-oncology. The first edition of this book, published in 1989, was of enormous value to physicians, nurses, and other health-care professionals in oncology because it presented a lucid cognitive behavioral therapy designed specifically for patients with cancer. The present volume retains the strengths of the earlier volume, and it extends and enriches those strengths based on advances that have been made in theory, research, and practice relevant to APT.

The pioneering research begun by Dr Greer in the 1970s provided keen insight into the psychological lives of people with cancer. The research showed that powerful patterns of coping can preserve the patient's sense of purpose and meaning even during the most dire phases of illness, while other patterns of coping can foster avoidance, fatalism, helplessness, and anxious preoccupation. Numerous studies showed the concurrent and longitudinal significance of these coping patterns in the psychological course of cancer.

Based on the findings of this research and on their own clinical experience, Dr Moorey and Dr Greer developed Adjuvant Psychological Therapy, a programme of cognitive behavioral therapy specifically for patients with cancer. In this volume, theory, research, and practice are presented in a manner that allows the reader to apprehend APT at multiple levels, ranging from the abstractions of formal cognitive theory to the specifics of questions and responses the therapist can use during the course of treatment.

Moorey and Greer's discussions of the cognitive bases of depression and anxiety and the emotional mechanisms associated with the regulation of specific emotion states are especially compelling. They also review relevant research thoroughly, giving the reader a sense of what therapies like APT have been shown to accomplish, and just as important, what they have been shown not to accomplish. The therapist's expectations for APT need to be realistic for the good of both the therapist and the patient, and the very balanced and thoughtful review of relevant research provides the basis for setting appropriate limits on these expectations. Thus the stage is well set for the clear, concrete guidance regarding cognitive, emotional, and behavioural therapeutic techniques that are described in subsequent chapters.

Those who work with oncology patients, or for that matter patients with any serious illness, often refer to the importance of spouses, adult children, or other family members who are closely involved with the patient. Usually, once this acknowledgment is made, little else is said. Fortunately, Moorey and Greer devote an entire chapter to this challenging topic. This aspect of care will continue increasing in importance as advances in the treatment of cancer that extend life continue to be made, and as health-care policies continue to shift care from hospital to home. They also treat end-of-life issues with great sensitivity, and describe how APT can increase well-being even at this stage of disease progression.

The volume benefits from Moorey and Greer's own impressive and extensive first-hand clinical experience with oncology patients. Examples from their respective practices are used effectively throughout the book to illustrate how APT looks and feels both to the therapist and the patient in the clinic setting. The examples also show how adaptive change can take place within a relatively short time, and how the therapist can help the patient recognize favourable change that might otherwise go undetected.

The second edition of *Cognitive behaviour therapy for patients with cancer* has a great deal to offer to a wide range of readers, including clinical researchers, therapists new to oncology, therapists practising other models of CBT, oncology nurses, hospice staff, social workers, and even patients themselves and their family members. The writing, as the authors intended, is free of jargon. Above all, the book's message is of central importance for anyone who cares about helping to maintain the psychological well-being of cancer patients and their family members. With this book, Moorey and Greer continue to lead the way in helping oncology patients and those around them maintain a sense of purpose, meaning, and well-being.

Susan Folkman, PhD
San Francisco
August 2001

Preface to the second edition

When the first edition of this book was published in 1989, Professor Tim McElwain—one of Britain's most eminent oncologists—wrote in the preface:

> Of course what we have here is very much a work in progress, and clearly there will be more to be done to refine, augment and validate the treatments advocated; but I feel certain that this important book will be of immediate value to everyone concerned with the management of cancer patients.

We have followed Professor McElwain's prescription by carrying out randomized trials of our treatment; these studies are reported in detail in the present edition. The whole field of psycho-oncology—in its infancy in 1989—has grown rapidly and we have included relevant studies here. Cognitive behaviour therapy has also changed in the last ten years, with the introduction of cognitive conceptualizations that take more account of developmental experiences and fundamental beliefs about the self and the world. The richer formulations that result are used in this new edition. Sections of the book have been rewritten or expanded and several new chapters have been added. We have kept the structure of the first edition. *Part One* covers some of the more important clinical, theoretical and empirical aspects of the psychology of cancer. It begins with an account of the experiences of people with cancer and the common emotional reactions to the disease. In the second chapter these reactions are put into a cognitive behavioural context, with an updated cognitive model of adjustment to cancer. Chapters 3 and 4 review the evidence for the effectiveness of cognitive behavioural interventions in people with cancer and for the impact of therapy on the disease process itself. *Part Two* is a manual of our version of cognitive behaviour therapy for cancer patients (Adjuvant Psychological Therapy). We begin this section with an overview of adjuvant psychological therapy followed by a description of the structure and the nature of the therapeutic relationship. Chapters 7–10 present the basic emotional, behavioural and cognitive techniques used in therapy. Chapter 11 describes how partners can be included in the therapy session. Chapter 12 addresses the special application of cognitive behaviour therapy to people with advanced disease or terminal illness, a challenging and rewarding area of work which has traditionally been more the preserve of humanistic and supportive therapies, and in Chapter 13 we describe the application of cognitive behavioural techniques to groups. We hope we have provided a book which is easily readable (i.e. as free of jargon as possible), informative and, above all, of immediate practical use for professionals involved in the clinical care of patients with cancer. This book should be of interest to nurses and oncologists who wish to learn how to apply a problem-focused approach to their patients' psychological concerns as well as to psychologists and psychiatrists working in medical settings. We hope, too, that our book will stimulate interest in the growing field of psycho-oncology.

We would like to thank Dr Katherine Mannix and Ms Mary Ward for their very helpful comments on an earlier draft of the text and to Mrs Kathleen Brennan and Laraine Pereira for their invaluable secretarial assistance. It is with sadness, that we record the deaths of Tim McElwain and of Teresa Gladwell our secretary and data manager. We are greatly indebted to them as well as to our patients who have taught us much.

Stirling Moorey
Steven Greer

Contents

PART ONE

The Psychology of Cancer

Chapter 1

What people with cancer feel

John was a 26-year-old bricklayer who led an active life, dividing his time between his girlfriend, his mates, and football (not necessarily in that order). He was a strong healthy man who enjoyed life and who had no previous history of serious physical or psychiatric illness. One day while making love his girlfriend noticed that his left testicle was swollen. She persuaded him to go to his doctor who referred him to an oncologist. He was found to have testicular cancer and that same evening, after writing suicide notes to his mother and girlfriend, he killed himself with a massive drug overdose.

The tragedy of this man's death was compounded by the fact that testicular germ-cell tumours in young adult men are highly curable (Horwich 1995). Fortunately, such tragic cases are rare, but they illustrate the strength of emotional distress that cancer can evoke.

Correct diagnosis is needed

There can be little doubt that in most people a diagnosis of cancer evokes a dread which is greater than that of other diseases carrying equally serious or worse prognoses (McIntosh 1974). Despite well-publicized progress in treatment, for many people the word *cancer* suggests a wild, uncontrollable proliferation of cells destroying the body and leading to a slow, painful death. Not surprisingly, therefore, doctors have until relatively recently shielded patients from learning the diagnosis. How do patients feel about this? To appreciate patients' feelings, imagine you are a patient who has developed cancer. Your doctor, believing that you cannot cope with the truth, will refuse to give you the correct diagnosis and fob you off with euphemisms. Your partner or close relative is told that you have cancer and advised on no account to reveal the diagnosis but to maintain a cheerful facade in front of you. Meanwhile, your symptoms grow worse, you begin to suspect that you might have cancer but neither your doctor nor your nearest and dearest will tell you the truth. You are told that you require an operation. You are admitted to a general surgical ward. There you become uneasily aware of an all too common practice; on ward rounds, the surgical team stand at the foot of your bed and discuss your case in low whispers, you observe that is not the case when dealing with other patients on the ward. Feeling isolated, increasingly anxious and helpless, you undergo major surgery. In that climate of fear and uncertainty, it is highly likely that you will feel intense emotional distress.

Experiences of this kind were common in the nineteen fifties and sixties. An American survey reported that as many as ninety per cent of doctors did not reveal the diagnosis of cancer to their patients (Oken 1961). This was also conventional practice in Britain. Doubtless, doctors who shielded patients from that dreaded diagnosis acted with the best intentions. But were they right? In what was a daring British pioneer study—given the climate of opinion at that time—a series of patients with cancer attending hospital for radiotherapy were told the diagnosis and their reactions were assessed one to four weeks later (Aitken-Swan and Easson 1959). The results were instructive: 66 per cent approved of having been told they had cancer, only 7 per cent disapproved and, interestingly, 19 per cent denied that they had been told (the reactions of the remaining 7 per cent could not be ascertained). That a majority of patients with cancer wanted to be informed of the diagnosis was a salient finding which began to bring about a change in medical attitudes and clinical practice. Although the practice of not revealing a cancer diagnosis to patients persists to this day in Southern and Eastern Europe, disclosure of the diagnosis is now common practice in Western Europe, North America, and Australia (Holland and Marchini 1998). But the change in medical attitudes is not confined to disclosing the diagnosis, welcome though that is. There has been a sea change from the paternalistic attitude adopted by many surgeons to a more evenly balanced professional relationship in which the patient is fully informed about her disease—or, rather, as informed as she wishes to be—and invited to take part in decisions regarding treatment. That at least, is what is supposed to have happened. In reality, the change has been slow in coming and is patchy throughout the UK. In the following account, a patient describes her experience (in 1998) to one of the authors:

> I started getting pains in my stomach and I thought it was just indigestion. Then I started getting constipated but sometimes diarrhoea as well. I began to go off my food. My husband made me go to the doctor who sent me to the hospital. They did some very unpleasant tests but never told me what it was. The surgeon asked me to wait outside while he spoke to my husband. All I could get out of either of them was that there was a bit of my bowel which wasn't right, and I had to have an operation and then some drugs afterwards. I began to worry that it was something serious—I couldn't get it out of my mind.
>
> I thought 'could it be the big C?' but when I finally plucked up the courage to ask, the surgeon just said: 'You mustn't worry yourself—it's a bit of bowel that isn't working properly and when we take it out you should be alright'. After the operation, I was given drugs which made me feel sick all the time. I lost my appetite, got more and more pain and just felt awful. I worried the whole time and used to cry a lot when on my own. My husband and daughter used to try to cheer me up by saying 'You'll get better soon' but after a while I didn't believe them anymore. I got more and more frightened and shaky and couldn't eat. I felt completely alone ... the worst part was not knowing, not being able to talk to anyone. It's funny, now that you have told me what's really wrong with me, I somehow feel stronger in myself. I know it's very serious and I'm still frightened, but not like before. I honestly feel better for knowing the truth ... it's such a relief to be able to talk about it.

Anxiety and depression

Giving patients the diagnosis, however, is not enough on its own. The traumatic impact of a cancer diagnosis requires close attention to the patient's emotional needs.

But since the advent of high technology medicine and increasingly narrow specialization, this important aspect of medical care has become relatively neglected. What patients feel when their emotional needs are ignored can be illustrated by their own comments:

A physician suffering from lymphoma:

Today's oncologists need to be encouraged to derive feelings of self-esteem and career satisfaction from improving the quality as well as the quantity of the patient's existence. By addressing the emotional problems associated with chemotherapy they can diminish their patient's feelings of abandonment and rage and prevent the despair which patients suffer…(Cohn 1982)

A patient with Hodgkin's disease:

… my experiences have taught me that adjusting to life with Hodgkin's disease has as much to do with emotional attitudes and communication as with physical states … while doctors still inquire 'How do you feel?', it seems to me that increasing reliance upon high technology diagnostic equipment has led to a decreasing emphasis on the importance of my reporting my body state. I came to resent this. (Cooper 1982)

Faced with a diagnosis of cancer, most people react initially with numbed shock and disbelief followed by anxiety, anger, and depression. In most cases, this stress reaction subsides within a few weeks as patients learn—painfully and slowly—to come to terms with their disease. Patients can be helped to make this adjustment by their doctor's sensitive, sympathetic counsel and by the emotional support of family and close friends. But a substantial minority go on to develop persistent psychological disorders. In our study of 1260 patients with various cancers attending the Royal Marsden Hospital, who were screened psychologically 4 to 12 weeks after an initial diagnosis of cancer 23 per cent were found to have clinically significant anxiety (15 per cent) or depression (8 per cent) (Greer et al. 1992). In addition, some patients who have coped well with the initial diagnosis are psychologically overwhelmed subsequently by the news that their cancers have recurred or spread. At the most conservative estimate, between 25 per cent and 30 per cent of patients suffer from cancer-related psychological disorders. If untreated, these disorders may persist for years even in the absence of any evidence of disease (Morris et al. 1977; Fobair et al. 1986; Irvine et al. 1991; Kornblith et al. 1992). As an example, a prospective study of an unselected series of patients with breast, lung, and colorectal cancers revealed that there was no improvement in psychological adaption over time. In fact, a significant decline in mental health scores between baseline assessment and 1–2 years after diagnosis was found (Ell et al. 1989).

In the early stages it may be treatment that causes most distress, rather than the effects of the disease itself. Surgery is often tolerated as a 'necessary evil' because it is seen as a treatment that will root the cancer out, but subsequent chemotherapy and radiotherapy can be more difficult to deal with, particularly if they are given as prophylactic treatments to patients who are otherwise feeling well. Mastectomy has been shown to be associated with high levels of anxiety and depression (Morris et al. 1977; Maguire et al. 1978; Grandi et al. 1987) with up to a quarter of women remaining depressed one year after the operation. But there seems to be a similar incidence of psychological morbidity in lumpectomy as well as mastectomy patients (Fallowfield 1986; van Heeringen *et al.* 1990). Between 25 and 50 per cent of colostomy patients experience psychological problems (Devlin *et al.* 1971; Wirsching *et al.* 1975; Eardley *et al.* 1976). High rates of depression and work problems were found in people who had undergone laryngectomy (Barton 1965; Drummond 1967).

Radiotherapy commonly causes nausea and fatigue (Peck 1972; Greenberg *et al.* 1992) and it may sometimes be difficult to distinguish these symptoms from the lethargy experienced in depressive reactions. Agitation, withdrawal, non-engagement with treatment and unrealistic expectations of treatment have been cited as predictors of poor outcome in radiotherapy (Schmale *et al.* 1982). In a recent study Montgomery *et al.* (1999) reported that 30 per cent of patients receiving radiotherapy suffered from adjustment disorder and/or anxiety/depression. Chemotherapy is also associated with high levels of anxiety and depression (40 per cent of patients in a study by Middelboe *et al.* 1995). The incidence of psychological problems may be lower when chemotherapy is given to produce symptomatic improvement, as in lung cancer (Hughes 1985) than when given as a prophylactic treatment.

Systematic studies of psychological morbidity among patients with cancer provide useful statistical data. Nothing, however, can convey what these patients really feel as vividly as their own descriptions. A 57-year-old man upon learning that he had developed lung cancer:

> At first I couldn't take it in, I didn't believe it … I went all numb, then I thought perhaps the doctors have made a mistake, you read about it all the time. But deep down I knew I had cancer … I was very, very scared at first, then I felt very low. I went into my shell, didn't want to see anyone; I couldn't tell my wife how I felt, I still can't.

A 36-year-old woman who had undergone a mastectomy, chemotherapy, and was put on long-term Tamoxifen. After 18 months, she was found to have a metastatic deposit in her sternum:

> It's hard to describe what I feel; fear, of course, utter misery, helplessness. It was bad enough the first time … I went through all that chemo and had my breast off and now it turns out it was all for nothing.

Disturbed relationships

In addition to anxiety and depressive states, patients have reported other difficulties in their lives particularly sexual dysfunction (e.g. Morris *et al.* 1977; Andersen 1986; Northouse *et al.* 1998). The effect of cancer on marital and other intimate relationships will depend in part on the quality of these relationships beforehand. The impact of cancer often exacerbates pre-existing problems. For instance, men who see illness as weakness, have a need to control others, or avoid confrontation find it harder to cope with their partner's breast cancer and this impairs marital interactions (Carter *et al.* 1993). On the other hand, previously close relationships are rarely damaged and may become even closer as the threat to life of cancer makes both partners realize how important they are to each other (Morris *et al.* 1977; Zucchero 1998). Good marital relationships can buffer the stress of cancer, and are associated with less psychological distress in the patient (Rodrigue and Park 1996).

Less well recognized than marital problems but no less important is the effect which breast cancer may have on the mother–daughter relationship (Lichtman and Taylor 1986; Wellisch *et al.* 1992; Zahlis and Lewis 1998). Mothers of adolescent daughters, in particular, have reported dramatic rejecting responses. In the words of one mother with breast cancer:

> My daughter went out of her way to make it harder for me. She would come in and she would make a mess in the kitchen, knowing that I couldn't clean it up. One night, she simply took off and left a note saying that she had to get out of the house. We didn't know where she was and I was completely hysterical. (Lichtman *et al.* 1985)

Sexual dysfunction

A common but insufficiently recognized complication of cancer is sexual dysfunction (Schover 1998). Sexual problems can be a consequence of cancer-related anxiety and depression or result from psychological and physical damage following certain treatments such as disfiguring surgery, ostomies, surgical nerve damage, radical pelvic irradiation, side-effects of chemotherapy and hormone treatment.

A 64-year-old man with a colostomy following surgery for cancer of the colon was referred for depression:

> To tell you the truth, doctor, I've been depressed since I had the operation last February (8 months ago). Don't think I'm not grateful to the surgeon, he did what he had to do, he cut out the cancer. It's just that I hate this bag so much; I can't get used to it. I'm frightened it will leak or smell. I don't go anywhere or do anything. [How does your wife feel about it?] Well … she's very good about it … but, to tell you the truth, … it's hard to say this, but I'm not a man anymore. That's made me feel worse than anything … I'm really sad about that. My wife says it doesn't matter, but I know it does. She's a lot younger than me; we've always had a good sex life. Now it's all gone. (He has tears in his eyes.)

A 42-year-old woman described her feelings one year after mastectomy:

> I'm not a complete woman anymore. My partner has tried to reassure me, but I feel so unattractive … I look horrible; I looked at the scar once and quickly turned away from the mirror. I've never looked at my chest since. When I have a bath I cover my top half up. I've never let Jim see me naked and we haven't made love since the operation. It's put a great strain on our relationship … Jim says he loves me and wants me, but I couldn't bear him to touch me there and see how ugly I am now.

In the literature on the complications of cancer treatments—with rare exceptions— sexual functioning is either ignored completely or given short shrift. It would appear that many clinicians consider it inappropriate to discuss sexual matters in the context of cancer, and many older patients, in particular, are too embarrassed to mention this topic. Such embarrassment can be overcome easily if clinicians routinely enquire about sexual function as part of their assessment of the quality of life of patients. It is important to obtain information about sexual dysfunction for two reasons: first, because such information will encourage the development of nerve-sparing surgical procedures, for example, replacing abdomino-perineal resection with low sphincter-saving resection for rectal cancer (Williams and Johnston 1983) and second, because effective treatment for sexual dysfunction is now possible in many cases (see Chapter 11).

Acute confusional states

So far we have described what are essentially chronic psychological disorders among patients with cancer. Acute disturbances, though less common, may also arise in the form of confusional states. Patients become restless, suspicious, noisy, angry, and confused with impaired concentration, memory and orientation for time and place. Their mood is usually abnormal, ranging from depression to euphoria. Acute confusional states are often worse at night. Opioid analgesics are the commonest cause; other causes include steroids, certain chemotherapeutic agents such as cis-platinum, interferon, vincristine, primary or secondary cerebral tumours and encephalopathy due to metabolic disturbances such as hypercalcaemia and electrolyte imbalance, carcinoid tumours, and paraneoplastic syndromes. Confusional states are particularly common in patients with advanced cancer. In about 50 per cent of cases, the cause of the confusional state cannot be determined (Bruera *et al.* 1990).

By far the commonest disorders are anxiety and depressive states attributable to the emotional impact of primary cancer and its recurrence. In practice, however, it is often difficult to separate the emotional impact of cancer from side-effects of treatment. An obvious example is the woman who develops breast cancer; the psychological trauma of learning that she has cancer may be compounded by mourning for the loss of the whole or part of her breast.

It is important to note that approximately two-thirds of patients with cancer do *not* develop chronic psychological disorders. It is a common clinical experience that two individuals with the same type and stage of cancer undergoing the same treatment will differ in their psychological responses. The following examples are typical:

> Betty, a 41-year-old married woman who worked as a computer operator, noticed a lump in her breast while taking a shower. She consulted her family doctor who referred her to an oncology unit where a diagnosis of breast cancer was made. After the initial shock of the diagnosis, she became anxious, sad, tearful, and found it difficult to get off to sleep. But three weeks later, following surgery and the commencement of chemotherapy and Tamoxifen, Betty's anxiety and depression subsided; she reported—and her husband confirmed—that she was coping well and back to her old self.

> Jane, 43, divorced, was a social worker. She too discovered a breast lump which turned out to be cancer. Like Betty, her cancer was at an early stage and had not spread; Jane received exactly the same treatment as Betty. Despite these similarities, Jane's psychological response to the diagnosis of cancer was quite different. She became increasingly anxious and preoccupied with fear that the cancer would return; she examined her body four or five times every day to check for lumps. She was tense, restless, and unable to lead a normal life because of intrusive thoughts about cancer; she complained of poor sleep and poor appetite. At least once a week, she consulted her family doctor requesting

reassurance that the cancer had not recurred. When first seen in the Department of Psychological Medicine, she had been in this depressed state for nearly four months.

Many such examples could be cited. What are the reasons for the individual differences in psychological response to cancer? This intriguing question has important clinical implications, for it leads directly to the possibility of designing effective psychological therapy. Our own work and that of others, especially Lazarus and Folkman's (1984) landmark studies of stress, indicate that an important determinant of any given patient's psychological response is how the threat of cancer is perceived (appraised) together with the particular coping skills which that person can use to reduce the threat. In this book, we examine this theme in some detail and describe the ensuing development of psychological therapy specifically designed for patients with cancer.

Chapter 2

A cognitive model of adjustment to cancer

The descriptions in the previous chapter of the different reactions of Betty and Jane to the diagnosis of breast cancer illustrate well the central role that meaning plays in adjustment to serious illness. Although both women had the same good prognosis, Betty felt able to cope but Jane did not. After an initial period of confusion and distress, Betty engaged actively in her treatment, believing she could deal with the problems that cancer posed and recover from the disease. Jane, on the other hand, was unable to get the cancer out of her mind. She was overwhelmed with the possibility that it might recur. Cognitive models of adjustment and coping all assume that it is the interpretations we make about stressful events that determine how we respond to them (Lazarus and Folkman 1984; Folkman and Greer 2000). Faced with cancer we may, like Betty, see the diagnosis as a challenge which we feel equipped to handle. Others, like Jane, may see it as such a huge threat, they do not have the resources to come through. Still others view the harm as already done; cancer is not seen as a threat but a death sentence.

Cancer threatens fundamental assumptions about our lives. Deeply held beliefs about ourselves, the world, and relationships suddenly come into question. If we have believed we are strong, how do we manage the debilitating effects of chemotherapy? If we have strongly valued our appearance, how do we now view ourselves after a mastectomy? What happens to our belief that the world is a benevolent and a just place? Some of the assumptions that are challenged by a diagnosis of cancer are universal. Some are very personal. We have found it useful to differentiate between the impact the disease has on beliefs about survival and beliefs about who we are.

The threat to survival

Although we may be aware that one in three of us will develop cancer at some time in our lives, we usually operate as if we are somehow immune. People generally see themselves as less likely than others to be victims of diseases, crimes, and accidents and have overly optimistic expectations about the future (Perloff 1983, 1987; Taylor and Armor 1996). Most of us have great difficulty imagining the end of our lives; as Freud wrote, it is 'impossible to imagine our own death; and whenever we attempt to do so we can perceive that we are in fact still present as spectators' (Freud 1953). Some researchers suggest that we normally have silent assumptions that we are both invulnerable and immortal (Janoff-Bulman 1999). We tacitly believe that the world is a just place and we are essentially in control. These assumptions are shattered by the diagnosis of cancer. The initial reaction to this diagnosis, as Greer (1985) remarked, is to view the diagnosis of cancer as a 'catastrophic threat tantamount to a death sentence'. The initial period after the diagnosis is marked by confusion and a chaotic jumble of thoughts and feelings. There is also usually a numbness, with times of great emotional turmoil alternating with a deadening of feelings ('This can't be happening to me'). From a cognitive perspective, this is the result of core beliefs about the self, the world, and the future being challenged. At first it is difficult to make sense of what is happening. In the weeks and months following a diagnosis of cancer, patients begin to answer three vital questions about what the illness means:

1 How great is the threat?
2 What can be done about it?
3 What is the prognosis?

The threat represented by a diagnosis of cancer can be interpreted in several ways (Fig. 2.1). It can be seen as a challenge, it can be seen as a major threat which can overwhelm or destroy, or it can be seen as harm, loss or defeat. A fourth possibility exists—denial or refusal to accept that the threat exists at all. The personal meaning of cancer for an individual will be an important factor in determining their adjustment to the disease.

Lazarus and Folkman (1984) have contributed greatly to our understanding of how people cope with stress by demonstrating the role of appraisals in the coping process. As well as this primary appraisal of the nature of the stress, a secondary appraisal takes place. This corresponds to our second question: What can I do about it? Patients vary in their beliefs about the extent to which they, or anyone, can control or alter the disease process. The answer to the third question (What is the prognosis?) arises from the answers to the first two questions. If the disease represents a challenge that can be met, the patient feels optimistic. If it is seen as a loss and the individual feels helpless in the face of it, then the future will look very bleak. The patterns of thoughts, feelings, and behaviours associated with these appraisals represent the style of adjustment the person develops.

Greer and Watson (1987) have identified five common adjustment styles:

+ Fighting spirit
+ Avoidance or denial

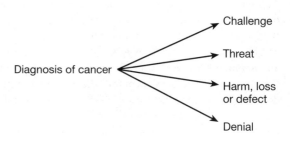

Fig. 2.1 The appraisal of the diagnosis of cancer.

- Fatalism
- Helplessness and hopelessness
- Anxious preoccupation.

Fighting spirit

The person sees the illness as a challenge, and has a positive attitude towards outcome. He or she engages in various behaviours such as seeking appropriate, but not excessive, information about the disease, taking an active role in his or her recovery, and attempting to live as normal a life as possible. The diagnosis is seen as a challenge, the individual can exert some control over the stress, and the prognosis is seen as optimistic. Typical statements of a patient with a fighting spirit might be:

'I don't dwell on my illness.'
'I try to carry on my life as I've always done.'
'I see my illness as a challenge.'
'I keep quite busy so I don't have to think about it.'

Avoidance or denial

The person denies the impact of the disease. The threat from the diagnosis is minimized and consequently the issue of control is irrelevant and the prognosis is seen as good. The attitude of denial is accompanied by behaviour which minimizes the impact of the disease on the patient's life. Patients make statements such as:

'They just took my breast off as a precaution.'
'It wasn't that serious.'

A more conscious form of this, which has been termed *positive avoidance*, is encouraged in adjuvant psychological therapy. This involves trying to get on with life without thinking about cancer and by using distraction.

Fatalism

The diagnosis represents a relatively minor threat, there is no control that can be exerted over the situation, and the consequences of lack of control can and should be accepted with equanimity. The patient has an attitude of passive acceptance. Active strategies towards fighting the cancer are absent. The person may make statements such as:

'It's all in the hands of the doctors/God/fate.'
'I've had a good life, what's left is a bonus.'

Helplessness and hopelessness

In this adjustment style, the patient is overwhelmed and engulfed by the enormity of the threat of cancer. The individual's focus of attention may be on the impending loss of life or on the illness as a defeat. The diagnosis is seen as a major threat, loss, or defeat, there is a belief that no control can be exerted over the situation, and the perceived negative outcome is experienced as if it has already come about. Active strategies for fighting the cancer are absent and there may be a reduction in other normal activities. Basically, the patient gives up. A person who is helpless and hopeless will say:

> 'There's nothing I can do to help myself.'
> 'What's the point in going on?'

Anxious preoccupation

Anxiety is the predominant affect in this adjustment style. The behavioural component is one of compulsive searching for reassurance. Much of the time is spent worrying about the disease coming back, and any physical symptoms are immediately identified as signs of new disease. Reassurance is sought by self-referral, use of alternative medicine, and excessive searching for information about cancer. The diagnosis represents a major threat, there is uncertainty over the possibility of exerting control over the situation, and the future is seen as unpredictable. Typical statements of the anxiously preoccupied patient are:

> 'I worry about the cancer returning or getting worse.'
> 'I have difficulty believing this happened to me.'
> 'I can't cope with not knowing what the future holds.'

Threat to survival and psychological adjustment

There is considerable evidence that attitude towards cancer is associated with overall psychological adjustment. Fighting spirit has been consistently shown to correlate with lower levels of anxiety and depression (Watson *et al.* 1988, 1990), women with breast cancer who have a greater perception of control over the disease show better adjustment (Taylor *et al.* 1984), and general optimism predicts distress over the year following surgery for breast cancer (Carver *et al.* 1993). In one interesting study female college students who scored highly on a measure of hope were asked to imagine how they would cope with cancer. They were both more knowledgeable about cancer and described more hope-specific coping responses than college students who were generally less hopeful (Irving *et al.* 1998). Cancer patients with a helpless–hopeless or anxiously preoccupied adjustment style are more likely to be depressed or anxious (Osborne *et al.* 1999).

The threat to the self

The possibility of death is the most serious threat that any of us could face, but this is by no means the only threat in cancer. The morbidity of the disease can sometimes prove more difficult to cope with than the fear of death. Symptoms of cancer may be painful and debilitating, like many other diseases, and treatment may also cause suffering. Figure 2.2 shows a schematic representation of the very real negative consequences of the diagnosis of cancer.

Symptoms of the disease and its treatment can be aversive in a variety of ways. They may cause pain, weakness and lethargy, nausea and vomiting, impaired concentration and impaired mobility. These can in turn produce severe disruption of the patient's lifestyle. Previously rewarding activities may need to be reduced or even abandoned, sometimes permanently. This does not just apply to specific activities, but may also require more general changes in role. Work may no longer be possible, and for

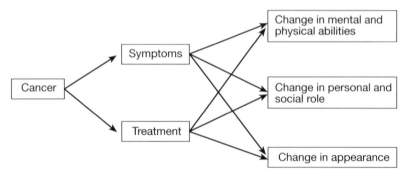

Fig. 2.2 Negative consequences of the diagnosis of cancer.

younger patients many of the demands of parenting may be too great. The results of physical disability and behavioural limitation can require adjustments of family roles on the part of the patient and of other family members. Even if the patient is relatively well, treatment sometimes has drastic effects on bodily appearance, ranging from the temporary hair loss of radiotherapy and chemotherapy (Maguire *et al.* 1980), to permanent change after surgical treatments (Morris *et al.* 1977; Maguire *et al.* 1978).

As with the threat of death, it is the appraisal of these consequences of cancer that contributes to the person's emotional reaction. Most, though by no means all, men can accept baldness as a side-effect of chemotherapy because being bald is a socially acceptable state for men. For women, for whom appearance is socially much more important, losing hair is a considerable threat to their self-image. Other consequences of cancer may play into more idiosyncratic belief systems, which do not fit cultural norms. For a woman to whom appearance is of central importance, the removal of a small tumour on the skin might cause extreme distress, even if the scarring was only minimal. For a man to whom work is the most important thing in life, a spell of three months' sickness could be catastrophic, even if he can be assured that the cancer will be cured. The threats that cancer poses to appearance, physical and mental ability, and to social role will therefore affect individuals differently depending on the meaning they give to them. What we have termed 'threats to the self' could also be called threats to the 'personal domain'. Beck (1976) has written extensively on the way in which 'a person's emotional response …depends on whether he perceives events as adding to, subtracting from, endangering or impinging upon his domain'. The personal domain refers to those aspects of his life—both tangible and intangible—which an individual sees as having direct relevance to himself, e.g. family, friends, possessions, values, goals. Silberfarb and Greer (1982) identified four common emotional reactions to cancer: anxiety, anger, guilt, and depression. The particular interpretations the patient makes about cancer give rise to these emotions, and they can be seen as interpretations of particular threats to the personal domain.

Anxiety

Key elements: danger and vulnerability These two themes are necessary to the individual's interpretation of a situation if he or she is to experience anxiety. Danger is present if the situation is seen as threatening to the person's physical or social well-being, whereas vulnerability results from the perception that the patient or other people will not be able to deal with the threat. In assessing risk we take account of how likely it is that the negative event will occur, as well as how bad it will be if it does occur. Even a low probability of recurrence can be intolerable if the consequences of recurrence are seen as awful and terrible. The resources available to deal with the threat will diminish anxiety. If we believe that oncologists can cure our cancer we will feel less anxious, but if we do not trust them the threat will increase. If we find it hard to have faith in our own coping abilities this will also increase our fear.

As we have seen, death is not the only thing that people with cancer fear. The possibility of physical impairment, disfigurement, or invalidity can be a source of great anxiety. Patients who have panic attacks may believe that the bodily symptoms they are experiencing signify impending madness. Mothers who are overprotective may become preoccupied with how their children will cope if they die, while overly self-reliant people may panic at the thought of the loss of control which their illness implies.

Anger

Key element: unjustified attack Anger is generated if the person believes his or her personal domain has been attacked in some way. This may be a direct attack on physical safety or on self-esteem, or it may be a more indirect attack on certain rules or values that the person holds dear. The angry person is concerned by the unjustness of the threat being faced, whereas the anxious person is more concerned by the possible effects of the threat on personal safety. A focus on future pain and inability to cope creates anxiety. If they think about the doctor's failure to control the pain or on life's unfairness in making them suffer, they are more likely to become angry. This sense that an agent—personal or impersonal—is abusing them seems to be one of the basic requirements for an angry reaction. People may get angry at God for his failure to save them, or at their spouse for not providing adequate support. Having the illness may lead them to identify with other people's suffering, allowing them to get angry over health service cuts or a child's death as if it affected them directly.

By focusing on external violations of his or her rights, the angry person is thinking less about personal vulnerability or imperfection. It is possible to become locked in an angry mode, and for this to provide a form of defence against some of the more unpleasant consequences of the disease itself. A woman who had hormone-dependent breast cancer made repeated complaints about not receiving treatments to which she felt she was entitled. These included hormonal treatments and counselling. It is likely that she was working on a rule such as: 'I am entitled to the best treatment available and if I do not get it, it is because it is being deliberately withheld'. Her hostile strategy had the effect of both mobilizing her energy to fight the disease and preventing her from focusing too closely on its effects.

The decision as to whether or not a belief is maladaptive is not an easy one, and cannot be made simply on the basis of it being irrational. In this woman's case, her anger could be seen as having both adaptive and maladaptive functions. In fact, some studies have supplied evidence that these 'hostile patients', who are often labelled as difficult by their doctors, survive longer than more compliant patients (Derogatis *et al.* 1979). On the other hand, a study by Taylor *et al.* (1984) indicated that women with breast cancer who blamed others had poorer psychological adjustment. Sadness and fear are socially acceptable emotions to relatives of patients, but anger presents more problems.

Guilt

Key element: self-blame The guilty person, like the angry one, is concerned with apportioning blame. An important rule has been violated, and someone is responsible. The difference is that the guilty person blames him- or herself. Guilt often exists as part of a depressive picture, but it may occur independently and when this happens it is often a result of the person's attempt to give meaning to his or her experience. In the search for an explanation for the illness, people with cancer may decide that they have brought it on themselves and are being punished for some sin or crime. If they can find some way of expiating their sin, or of gaining control over the disease, they may be able to overcome the guilt. If, however, they are unable to do this they may become fixated on the past and ruminate over the way they have ruined their life; 'If only I hadn't done that, I might not have become ill'. Thoughts such as 'I'm a burden' or 'I've brought this on my family' result in guilt and self-reproach about the effect of cancer on others. If the person with cancer has a rule that they are responsible for what people close to them feel or that it's their job to prevent their family feeling unhappy, they may feel guilty about having cancer. Rather than blaming the disease for the family's suffering, the person with cancer may unfairly blame him- or herself.

Sadness and depression

Key element: loss or defeat The theme of sadness is loss from the personal domain. The losses in cancer are self-evident—loss of parts of the body, loss of strength and vitality, loss of a valued role. The real losses that occur as a result of the objective consequences of the disease only cause a depressed mood if they are perceived as important by the patient. Loss of hair is not significant to someone who gives little value to physical appearance, and the opportunity to give up work may be welcomed by some people. It is only if the loss impinges on the personal domain that it produces sadness. If these reactions become enduring ways of viewing the self they become integrated into the person's self-concept.

Information processing in cancer

Once a negative view of the disease and its impact on the individual has established itself it tends to be self-perpetuating. Normally we have a slight selective bias for positive information. Taylor (Taylor and Armor 1996) suggests that when a person faces negative or threatening events, these positive assessments of self, personal control, and optimism about the future are challenged. An attempt is made to restore or enhance these positive perceptions leading to 'positive illusions' in the face of adversity. For instance, patients with heart disease and AIDS tend to compare themselves with patients they see as less fortunate than themselves (Helgeson and

Taylor 1993; Taylor *et al.* 1993). People with a fighting spirit may be more optimistic about their prognosis than is appropriate in the circumstances; this might be interpreted as choosing to see the glass as half full rather than half empty, and not an *illusory* view of their situation. The tendency to put the most positive spin on the implications of cancer for self-perception, self-control, and view of the future is usually associated with better adjustment, and a more active coping style (Taylor and Armor 1996). Although there may be a confirmatory positive bias present in people with good psychological adaptation, there certainly seems to be a negative bias in those showing maladaptive adjustment styles. Their negative schemata process information in such a way as to maintain their negative view of themselves or their survival. People with cancer who become depressed or anxious distort information in a similar way to other depressed or anxious patients. Numerous studies have demonstrated this cognitive bias (for a review of this literature see Clark and Steer 1996). The process of distorting this information in a negative way often involves systematic logical errors or cognitive distortions; the commonest of these have been identified by Beck (Beck *et al.* 1979) and are described below.

All-or-nothing thinking

Events are seen as black and white, with no shades of grey. For instance, a person may conclude that because his cancer cannot be cured, he might as well give up and die. The disease is perceived as cure or death, whereas the reality might be months or years of remission. An athletic person might conclude: 'If I'm not well enough to play football, I can get no pleasure from anything'.

Selective abstraction

A person may select part of the information available to suit his or her predominant cognitive set. When having a treatment explained, an anxious person may hear that it is painful and unpleasant but will pay less attention to the fact that it has a high chance of being successful. The depressed person with breast cancer focuses on the loss of her breast but pays little attention to the fact that her husband still finds her sexually attractive.

Arbitrary inference

The uncertainty of cancer prognosis means that there is often insufficient evidence on which to base judgements about the future. Patients may still come to arbitrary conclusions that the disease will inevitably recur and kill them. As well as jumping to conclusions, people make arbitrary inferences about other people's thoughts and motivations (mindreading). Harmless looks are interpreted as indicating that the relative knows something bad but will not disclose it.

Overgeneralization

In this distortion a single negative event is seen as a never-ending pattern. For instance, on her return from hospital a woman with ovarian cancer has her first argument with her husband. She says to herself: 'We'll never stop arguing, our marriage is over'.

Labelling

Labelling ignores the fact that people are complex mixtures of characteristics. Instead, it defines them in terms of a single global construct. Statements like: 'I'm just a chronic invalid' or: 'Nurses are angels' indicate that labelling is taking place.

Magnification and minimization

In this distortion, certain pieces of the perceptual field are enlarged or reduced in perspective to suit the person's cognitive set. In depression, for instance, the chances of a remission from the cancer might be minimized in the person's mind. Someone who is denying her problems will minimize the seriousness of symptoms—'they only took my breast off as a precaution'—whereas an anxious person might magnify the pain of an injection.

These thinking errors cause the person with cancer to misinterpret or bias his or her judgements about the disease. In people with a maladaptive adjustment style these processing biases produce *negative automatic thoughts*. These are idiosyncratic, plausible thoughts which come into consciousness unbidden. They contain logical errors in their reasoning, but to the person experiencing them they seem accurate and realistic. It is often only when the individual is removed from the stressful situation that these thoughts can be seen to be irrational. Typical automatic thoughts include:

> 'I can *never* be happy again.'
> 'It's no good fighting, you *always* get knocked for six.'
> 'I can't cope.'
> 'I hate myself.'
> 'The doctors only want to use me as a guinea-pig.'
> 'I'm not a real man/woman anymore.'

An automatic thought is a thought or an image which is not necessarily at the centre of the person's attention, but is accessible to consciousness. These thoughts, together with the emotions and behaviours with which they are associated, are the key components of cognitive behaviour therapy. Psychodynamic therapies make interpretations and inferences about unconscious processes. Cognitive therapies make use of conscious cognitions. Dreams may be the royal road to the unconscious, but thoughts give entry to the rules and meaning systems which govern our feelings and actions.

Thoughts, feelings, behaviour, and physiology

The discussion so far has given cognition a central place in adjustment to cancer. The view a person takes of the meaning of cancer directly influences their emotional and behavioural reactions, particularly their attempts at coping, but the relationship is not simply in one direction. There is a complex interplay between thoughts, feelings, behaviour and physical reactions in which no single component has primacy. For instance, thoughts like 'What's the point? I'm never going to get through this. It's hopeless' will increase a person's feelings of depression, but will also decrease motivation so that the person gives up social activities. With less chance to meet friends and

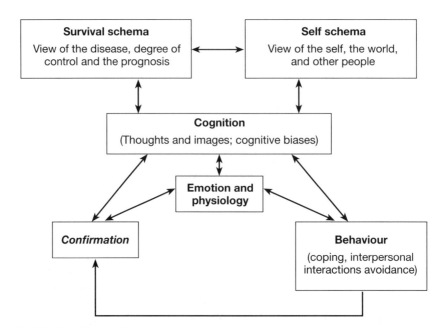

Fig. 2.3 Cognitive model of adjustment to cancer.

relatives there is more time for negative thinking, less pleasure and so the hopeless thoughts are confirmed and the mood becomes even lower. Depressed mood is often associated with fatigue and lethargy. These physical symptoms can be misinterpreted as evidence that the disease is worsening, reinforcing hopelessness and depression. Chapter 4 considers how mental processes may have a direct effect on the progression of cancer.

The role of family and friends

The interaction of the person with cancer with other people influences both the impact of the effects of the disease and his or her ability to cope with them. Family relationships can be dramatically changed as a result of the disease. The affected spouse may have to give up the role of caregiver, breadwinner, or supporter in the family. This may have wider implications for the quality of the family relationship.

The effects of the real changes brought about by the illness will again be determined by the personal meanings they hold for the all the actors in the drama. So it is not only the meaning of pain, debility and role change for the person, but also for other family members. Thus a complex interaction between the disease and members of the family, as well as between the family members themselves, is set up.

Much interest has been generated by the idea that social support can buffer the patient against some of the stresses of cancer. Some workers have predicted that patients with a wider social network or one that provides better emotional support will be better adjusted to the disease, and there does seem to be some evidence for this

(Helgeson and Cohen 1996). The evidence that exists on this is contradictory, but it may be the extent and quality of perceived support, not the objective level of support, that matter (Bloom 1986). Recent research has addressed the interactions between support and other factors. There may in fact be a reciprocal relationship between social support and adjustment. Psychological distress is related to decreased partner emotional support over time (Brady and Hegelson 1999) and women with high depression burden consistently lost more network members than did women who experienced depression but did not rank it among the top five side-effects of cancer (Badger *et al.* 1999).

Family members' ability to provide emotional support depends upon their own reaction to the disease. On the one hand, a husband who is so frightened by the thought of cancer that he believes nothing can be done to help will be ineffectual in helping his wife to fight the disease, whereas on the other hand, one who believes that patients must be cared for and should not be expected to do anything would also limit his wife's ability to function well. Renneker (1982) describes a husband who believed so strongly that cancer was incurable that he went out of his way to prevent his wife getting treatment that might have been curative.

It might be predicted that it is the partner's thoughts about cancer and the patient's role in the family which determine his or her emotional response. Coursey *et al.* (1975) found that anxiety is often greater in immediate family members than in patients themselves. Partners go through the same reactions to cancer as the patients, but their need to provide support often prevents them from being able to express their feelings openly. During treatment the patient may no longer be able to carry out his or her normal role and the stresses on the partner may consequently be great. Sometimes this results in observable depression or anxiety in the spouse, but more commonly it shows itself as problems in the relationship.

> A patient with lung metastases from breast cancer had always been the dominant partner. Her increasing breathlessness and disability threw her husband into a panic. He compensated by becoming the perfect nurse, constantly at her bedside, seeing to her every need. But periodically his own need for dependence would emerge and he collapsed. This resulted in his wife resuming her dominant role briefly, until the cycle repeated itself. This unsatisfactory state of affairs continued until her death.

Partners may also try to cope with stress by clinging to patterns of behaviour used before the cancer, refusing to alter their habits and pretending nothing has changed.

> The husband of one woman with breast cancer habitually reacted to stress and conflict by avoiding and ignoring it. He refused to visit her in hospital. When his wife came home he made no allowances for her illness, expecting her to look after the house and the children as before. Although she was not seriously physically ill, she felt tired and frightened. His inability to face the illness meant that she had no one to help her shoulder her emotional burden. In addition he expected her to carry on with no change in her daily routine, despite her fatigue.

Another type of problem arises when the illness upsets the balance of power or sharing of responsibility in the relationship. Resentment can occur on both sides as a result of this upset.

The effect of cancer on sexual function has already been described. People with cancer often think of themselves as less sexually attractive or, more subtly, see themselves as less potent or less feminine. These problems are compounded if communication difficulties ensue. A common example of this is seen with the husband who does not initiate lovemaking after his wife's mastectomy because he is not sure that she is well enough. If he does not give his reasons, the wife may misinterpret his behaviour as a sign that he no longer finds her attractive. When he does show an interest in sex she rebuffs him, hurting his feelings and reducing the likelihood that he will initiate further lovemaking.

Changes in the disease may exacerbate existing marital difficulties. These too can be understood in cognitive terms. Couples often operate on the basis of unrealistic rules or beliefs about each other. For instance, a person might believe that: 'My partner should know what is important to me without my having to tell him or her'. The onset of illness throws this system into stark relief, since there are now many new feelings and symptoms which the spouse is expected immediately to know about and be able to read in the patient. People close to the patient, particularly partner and family, but also doctors and nurses, have significant effects on their emotional state. Interaction with strangers and acquaintances can be nearly as important in some cases. In a study assessing the thoughts evoked by being in a situation with a disabled person whom one does not know well, Fichten (1986) found that anxiety was high, negative thoughts about the other person were prominent and self-efficacy beliefs were low compared with an interaction with an able-bodied person. Similar processes probably occur when healthy people meet others with cancer, particularly those with an obvious health disability. Feelings of embarrassment and discomfort can lead to reduced contact with an acquaintance who has cancer, resulting in increasing social isolation.

It is remarkable how well many relatives cope with the burdens cancer places on them. In some cases marriages may actually improve as a result of one partner having cancer (Hinton 1981; Hughes 1987), and despite the enormous strains, the divorce rates for long-term survivors do not seem to be higher than for the normal population (Fobair *et al.* 1986). The cognitive model must, then, take account of interpersonal factors which influence the individual's reaction. Interactions with family, friends, professionals, and strangers can all be significant. A series of interactions occur between the person and others that affect the person's perceptions of the real consequences of the disease as well as his or her ability to cope. This is a flexible and fluid process. Changes in any part of the system, whether it is deterioration in physical health or difference in the degree of support received, inevitably have effects on the other components. It is the way in which these changes are actively, cognitively processed that determines the final psychological reaction. In Chapter 11 we will show how this theoretical framework has been used to construct a psychological treatment for couples who face the stresses of cancer.

Vulnerability to adjustment disorders

Although cognitive behaviour therapy is primarily focused on the individual's reaction to the threats posed by cancer in the present, it does not ignore the influence of past experience on current appraisal and coping processes. Our fundamental beliefs about the world are formed from childhood experiences. If our parenting is good we will usually develop a sense that others are helpful and supportive, that the world is a relatively benign place where we can exert some control, and that we are worthwhile. As Janoff-Bulman (1999) points out, these beliefs are irrevocably changed by traumatic experience. Most people are able to adapt their world-view in the light of this new experience so that they see the world as both benign and potentially dangerous. Even some time after traumatic events, survivors' assumptions are less positive than those of the general population (Janoff-Bulman 1992). The more rigid and absolute these beliefs about a just and controllable world, the more difficult it will be to incorporate traumatic events into the world-view, or schema. This may lead to a sudden shift to a set of beliefs that the world is unjust and uncontrollable, and the development of the maladaptive adjustment styles already described.

Cognitive psychologists, building on the work of Bartlett (1932), have used the concept of a schema as a means of understanding how mental processes make sense of the world and make plans for action. A schema can be defined as: 'a relatively enduring structure that functions like a template; it actively screens, codes, categorizes and evaluates information. By definition it also represents some relevant prior experiences' (Kovacs and Beck 1978). The threat of cancer challenges schemas relating to a person's very existence and basic beliefs about himself, and the person is forced to modify or develop a new set of beliefs.

Not all core beliefs are positive to begin with. Alongside experiences of being loved and valued, most of us have had negative events in our lives that have led us to doubt our worth, our competence and our trust in others. If the experience of having cancer confirms these hidden doubts, a dormant negative schema may be activated. For instance, if a man witnessed constant arguments and violence between his parents as a child, he might develop a basic belief that the world is a chaotic and unpredictable place where bad things happen. Over the course of his life, however, he may develop a coping strategy of establishing control, elaborating a secondary belief that if he can control his life, he will be safe. The unpredictability of cancer threatens this fragile coping strategy and his core beliefs about the world will resurface, leading to the development of helplessness/ hopelessness or anxious preoccupation. Other cognitive therapists have developed similar models linking past experiences, underlying beliefs and people's reactions to illness (Liese 1993; Williams 1997; White 2001).

The clinical relevance of the cognitive model is expanded in part two of this book. The next two chapters will review the research relating to adjustment styles and the effectiveness of psychological therapy for cancer patients.

Summary

- Cancer is a life-threatening disease which poses a severe threat to many aspects of a person's life.
- It is not the objective consequences of the disease *per se* but the way in which they are interpreted that determine the individual's reactions.

- Emotional reactions are determined by the particular threat that cancer represents to the individual's personal domain. Core positive beliefs about the self, the world, and others are challenged, and core negative beliefs activated.
- The content of emotional reactions can be understood in terms of the cognitive processes which are taking place.
- The individual's adjustment to the disease is a result of the interaction between the interpretation of the stresses involved and the coping strategies available.
- The individual's adjustment to the disease is influenced by the quality of available emotional support.

Chapter 3

Can cognitive behaviour therapy improve quality of life?

There is now a considerable body of evidence concerning the effectiveness of psychological therapy in people with cancer. This ranges from clinical case reports and single case studies to large, well-designed, randomized controlled trials. Evaluating this evidence poses some problems, because the studies have not all asked the same research questions and the target patient populations may differ in various respects, so direct comparisons are not always possible. In fact, the question 'Can cognitive behaviour therapy improve quality of life?' proves to be too general. Most trials have looked at anxiety and depression and adjustment to the disease as indicators of quality of life, but other factors like interpersonal and social functioning have been less closely investigated. A psychological therapy could have more of an effect on some of these factors but not others. Aspects of the disease and the patient group could also influence the effectiveness of therapy. Many studies have used a mixed sample of cancer patients. This design can obscure differential effects of treatment on different diagnostic groups and it is only possible to do an analysis of subgroups if the sample is large. For instance, Edgar *et al.* (1992) found that the superiority of an early intervention over a late one which applied to the whole sample, did not apply for patients with breast cancer. When a single diagnostic group is investigated, it may be difficult to generalize findings to other groups. A second important variable is level of psychological distress. Most studies have taken all patients without selecting for psychological morbidity. However, there seems to be evidence that psychological therapy is of more benefit to people who are in a state of distress (Sheard and Maguire 1999). Side-effects of treatment and stage of disease could also influence the effects of psychological therapy. Therapy might well be helpful for people with early stage disease and a good prognosis but not for people with terminal illness. Because studies have taken various cancer diagnoses and intervened at different stages of the disease they cannot be compared easily and conclusions at the moment are tentative. With the exception of certain research groups that have carried out a systematic programme of investigation (e.g. Fawzy and colleagues, Cunningham and colleagues, and Greer and colleagues) most reports are of one-off trials, so our knowledge of the area is being built up in a relatively piecemeal fashion.

Because our intervention is a cognitive behavioural treatment (CBT) we will focus mainly on the evidence for the effectiveness of CBT. In this review, only randomized controlled trials of treatment have been included.

Individual cognitive behaviour therapy

Weissman and Worden (Weissman *et al.* 1980) were among the first to research psychological treatment in people with cancer systematically. Initially, they devised a psychological screening instrument that predicted emotional distress (Weissman and Worden 1977) and then assessed patients with newly diagnosed cancers of the breast, colon, lung, female reproductive tract, Hodgkin's disease, and malignant melanoma. One third of the patients (125) were found to be at high risk of emotional distress, but only 59 were eventually given psychological treatment, since 28 refused to participate and 38 were excluded on other grounds.

The patients were then allocated randomly to four sessions of consultation therapy or cognitive skills training. Consultation therapy consisted of helping people to identify problems, encouraging the ventilation of feelings associated with these problems, and exploring ways of solving the problems, preferably by direct confrontation. Emphasis was placed on the patient's personal control and competence. This patient-centred individualized approach was compared with cognitive skills training, that focused on the general process of psychosocial problem solving. The therapist first taught a step-by-step approach to problem solving by means of paired cards which depicted cancer-related problems and how these could be solved. Patients practised this approach and learned how to apply it to their own specific problems. Cognitive skills training also included relaxation training. Patients received homework assignments related to relaxation and problem solving. Both of these therapies had elements found in adjuvant psychological therapy (APT): cognitive skills training included structure and specific CBT techniques; consultation therapy contained problem solving, emotional expression, and enhancement of personal control.

Patients in the treatment group were compared with those from an untreated control group of patients from an earlier study who were at high risk of emotional distress. When assessed 2–6 months after diagnosis the two psychological treatments were equally effective in relieving emotional distress and improving psychosocial problem solving. This trial was a groundbreaking example of psychosocial research in oncology, in its development of a screening instrument for emotional distress, its detailed description of therapy, random allocation to treatment, and its use of an untreated control group. However, there were two methodological shortcomings:

◆ The untreated control group was obtained from an earlier study and therefore was not randomly allocated.

◆ Less than 50% of the study sample (*n*=125) actually took part in the treatment trial (*n*=59).

Linn *et al.* (1982) investigated the impact of counselling on adjustment in men with cancer who were judged to have a life expectancy of 3–12 months. Patients were randomly assigned to treatment or a no treatment control. Although not designated CBT, counselling included a mixture of non-directive and cognitive behavioural strategies similar to those used in APT. Therapists set out to reduce denial but maintain hope, to encourage meaningful activities, reinforce accomplishments, and increase self-esteem. In keeping with the late and often terminal stage of cancer treated in this study, the therapy commonly involved *being with* as much as *doing to* the patient: 'simply listening, understanding, and sometimes only sitting quietly with the patient were elements of treatment ... the therapist was often with the patient at the time of death'. Three months after the beginning of counselling the treated patients were less depressed, had higher self-esteem and an increased internal locus of control in comparison with the untreated controls.

Using an interesting study design, Edgar *et al.* (1992) compared CBT delivered early with CBT delivered later in the first year after diagnosis. Two hundred and five patients with various cancers were contacted as soon after diagnosis as possible and randomly allocated to an early intervention group which received treatment immediately or a late intervention group which received treatment 4 months later. The early intervention group began therapy on average 11 weeks after diagnosis, the late group 28 weeks after diagnosis. The intervention consisted of five sessions of 1 hour duration with a nurse. Techniques used included problem-solving, goal setting, cognitive reappraisal, and relaxation training. A multi-disciplinary workshop on the effective use of resources was also offered to patients at 4-month intervals.

Four months after diagnosis (when the early intervention group had received treatment but the late intervention group had not) there were no differences between the conditions. Eight months after diagnosis the late intervention group was significantly less depressed, anxious, and worried. At the 12-month assessment the late intervention group had less worry related to illness, but there were no other differences between treatments. Unfortunately this trial did not include a treatment as usual group, so we do not have a picture of the natural course of adjustment, and so do not know if the two methods of treatment delivery had any long-term advantage over no treatment. It would, from these results, appear that giving CBT later rather than sooner in the first year after diagnosis reduces distress more rapidly (although an analysis of subgroups showed that breast cancer patients did equally well in both conditions). The authors speculated that the emotional work that needs to be accomplished after diagnosis is too overwhelming to allow patients to benefit from coping skills training during the first few months. They suggest that if this approach is offered in the first few months, it may need to be continued longer until the patient can use the coping strategies. An alternative might be to incorporate more emotion-based work into the traditional CBT framework as we have done in APT (see Chapter 7).

Elsesser *et al.* (1994) conducted a small study which compared a combination of anxiety management and stress inoculation training with a waiting list control in people with various cancer diagnoses. There were slight improvements on psychological variables in the treatment group.

Randomized controlled trials of adjuvant psychological therapy

The first evaluation of our own treatment was a prospective randomized controlled trial comparing adjuvant psychological therapy with treatment as usual (Greer *et al.* 1992). Patients aged between 18 and 74 who were attending the Royal Marsden Hospital at the time of diagnosis or first recurrence of cancer were screened for psychological morbidity. To ensure a large enough sample for follow-up only people with a life expectancy of at least 12 months were eligible. The participants completed the Hospital Anxiety and Depression Scale (HAD) and the Mental Adjustment to Cancer Scale (MAC). Those who scored 10 or higher on the anxiety scale of the HAD, 8 or higher on the depression scale or who scored high on helplessness/hopelessness and low on fighting spirit on the Mental Adjustment to Cancer Scale were invited to take part in the study. Those who agreed to participate were randomly allocated to either six sessions of APT or a no treatment control. Those in the control group were able to access the usual support of the hospital but did not receive the structured intervention. The main outcome measures were the Hospital Anxiety and Depression Scale, Mental Adjustment to Cancer Scale, Rotterdam symptom checklist, and the psychosocial adjustment to illness scale. Assessments were made before therapy, at eight weeks, and at four months of follow-up. One hundred and seventy four patients entered the trial, of whom 156 (90%) patients completed the eight week trial; follow-up data at four months were obtained for 137 patients (79%). At eight weeks, patients receiving therapy had significantly higher scores than control patients on fighting spirit and significantly lower scores on helplessness, anxious preoccupation, and fatalism; anxiety; psychological symptoms; and on orientation towards health care. At four months, patients receiving therapy had significantly lower scores than controls on anxiety; psychological symptoms; and psychological distress. Clinically, the proportion of severely anxious patients dropped from 46% at baseline to 20% at eight weeks and 20% at four months in the therapy group and from 48% to 41% and to 43% respectively among controls. The proportion of patients with depression was

Table 3.1 Percentages of patients scoring more than 10 on the anxiety scale of the HADS in therapy and control groups

Assessment	APT	No treatment control
Baseline	46%	48%
8 weeks	20%	43%
4 months	20%	41%
1 year	19%	44%

Table 3.2 Percentages of patients scoring more than 8 on the depression scale of the HADS in therapy and control groups

Assessment	APT	No treatment control
Baseline	40%	30%
8 weeks	13%	19%
4 months	18%	23%
1 year	11%	18%

40% at baseline, 13% at eight weeks, and 18% at four months in the therapy group and 30%, 29%, and 23% respectively in controls. At 1 year there was a significant difference in change from baseline on the Psycholosocial Adjustment to Illness Scale and a tendency for the therapy group to show more change on measures of helplessness and anxiety (Moorey *et al.* 1994). Only 19% of therapy patients were in the clinical range for anxiety compared to 44% of the controls.

A striking feature of this study was the high refusal rate. When the reasons for this were examined it emerged that patients with stage I disease were most likely to refuse to participate. Patients were less likely to participate if they had low volume disease, were receiving no further treatment, or had fewer physical symptoms. Men who scored high on anxious preoccupation were more likely to agree to take part in the study.

Having demonstrated that APT was more effective than a 'treatment as usual' control, the next step was to compare the therapy with a control treatment in a clinical setting (Moorey *et al.* 1998). Patients were selected from the Psychological Medicine Clinic at the Royal Marsden Hospital. Patients with various cancers referred for psychiatric assessment, and who met criteria for an abnormal adjustment reaction, were randomly allocated to either 8 weeks of adjuvant psychological therapy, or 8 weeks of a comparison treatment of supportive counselling. Both treatments were administered by ourselves. The supportive counselling (like APT was conducted as individual weekly sessions, including the spouse where appropriate) was designed to control for therapist's time and attention and non-specific factors, but to exclude techniques thought to be key ingredients of APT. Non-directive techniques were used to encourage ventilation of feelings in an empathic therapeutic relationship. Information about cancer and the nature of emotional reactions to cancer was given if requested by the patient, or if the need arose during the session. The counselling sessions were unstructured with no agenda. Behavioural and cognitive techniques were not used, and no homework was assigned between sessions. Because both therapists had a strong allegiance to CBT and neither were trained Rogerian therapists, this cannot be considered a full comparison of APT with another therapy. However, we believe this approach approximates to the routine counselling many distressed people with cancer might receive from nurses and other professionals.

Similar outcome measures were used as in the first study. In addition to the HAD and the MAC scale, patients completed a measure of the types of coping strategies taught in APT (the Cancer Coping Questionnaire; CCQ). Some other measures, used more commonly in CBT for anxiety (the Spielberger State Trait Anxiety Inventory; Spielberger *et al.* 1970) and depression (the Beck Depression Inventory; Beck *et al.* 1961) were included so that comparisons with other CBT studies could be made.

At 8 weeks from the baseline assessment, APT had produced a significantly greater change than the counselling intervention on fighting spirit, helplessness, coping with cancer, anxiety, and self-defined problems. At 4 months from baseline, APT had produced a significantly greater change than counselling on fighting spirit, coping with cancer, anxiety and self-defined problems. Unfortunately, insufficient numbers of patients were available at follow-up (due to ill health or patients having moved away). These results are encouraging since they show that APT does not simply exert its effect through non-specific factors. The change in CCQ scores in CBT but not in counselling confirm that patients do learn to think in cognitive terms and to use strategies from the therapy.

Moynihan *et al.* (1998) evaluated adjuvant psychological therapy in men with testicular cancer. Whereas the first trial had taken patients with any cancer who were psychologically distressed, this trial focused on a single diagnostic group and assessed whether or not APT could help all patients—distressed or not. Patients attending the Testicular Tumour Unit at the Royal Marsden Hospital were randomly allocated to six sessions of APT or a treatment as usual control. Seventy-three of 184 (40%) eligible patients agreed to take part and 81 (44%) did not wish to participate but agreed to complete further assessments. Thirty patients wanted no further contact with the assessors. Only results for the Hospital Anxiety and Depression Scale were reported. At 2 months change from baseline favoured the treated group on the anxiety subscale, but this was not sustained when adjusted for factors related to the disease. By 12 months change from baseline seemed to favour the control condition. The authors concluded that men with testicular cancer seem to have considerable coping abilities, and that routine psychological support was not indicated.

Psychoeducational groups

Heinrich and Schag (1985) compared a psychoeducational programme for patients and their spouses with current available care. Four hundred and ninety four patients were screened and 92 met the screening criteria (Karnofsky score >70, age 25–70, no severe cognitive deficits, no serious psychiatric illnesses, living within 50 miles of the hospital). Eighty-one of these patients were contacted, and 70 eventually entered the study. Only 51 patients completed the pre- and post-evaluations. Most of the patients had been living with cancer for over two years. Therapy consisted of a structured small group programme. The goal of the group was to educate patients and spouses about cancer and its impact and to teach coping skills. The groups included education and information about cancer, relaxation training, modifications of Weissman and colleagues (1980) cognitive therapy, problem solving, and activity management. Activity management included a walking exercise component and contracting for patient and spouse to increase positively valued individual and couple activities.

Both groups improved over the course of the study and there were no significant differences on measures of adjustment. Patients and their spouses showed improvement on scores on the Cancer Information Test indicating that the educational component of the treatment had been successful. At the post-evaluation and 2 month follow-up there was a positive effect on coping in medical situations and achieving goals in the treated group. Both partners reported that the education and relaxation training were the most helpful components of the therapy. Although this intervention was targeted at spouses as well as patients, only 12 spouses in the treatment group and 13 in the control group completed the study (out of a possible 51).

Telch and Telch (1986) randomized 41 out-patients with a variety of cancer types and stages to one of three groups: coping skills instruction, supportive therapy, and no treatment control. The coping skills condition consisted of six sessions of

Table 3.3 Randomized controlled trials of individual cognitive behaviour therapies in cancer

Study	Interventions	n	Cancer type	Stage of disease	Selection	Outcome	Follow-up
Linn et al. 1982	Counselling v. no treatment	120	Men with various cancers	Advanced. Life expectancy 3–12 months	All patients	CBT>NTC	None
Weissman et al. 1980	4 sessions comparing 2 CBT interventions: Cognitive skills training (CST) v. consultation therapy (CT)	59	Various cancers	Newly diagnosed	Patients at high risk of emotional distress	2–6 months after diagnosis CST=CT	None
Edgar et al. 1992	5 sessions coping skills training administered early (EI) or late (LI)	205	Various cancers	Newly diagnosed	All patients	EI=LI at 4 months	8 months LI>EI; 1 year LI>EI; Worry
Greer et al. 1992; Moorey et al. 1994	6 sessions APT v. treatment as usual	156	Various cancers	Newly diagnosed and recurrence	Screened patients high in anxiety or depression	CBT>NTC	1 year CBT>NTC
Elsesser 1994	6 sessions Anxiety management training and Stress inoculation training	27	Various cancers	All stages	All patients	CBT>NTC; Effect only small	None

(continued)

Table 3.3 (continued) Randomized controlled trials of individual cognitive behaviour therapies in cancer

Study	Interventions	n	Cancer type	Stage of disease	Selection	Outcome	Follow-up
Fawzy et al. 1996	6 sessions group CBT v. individual CBT v. assessment only	104	Malignant melanoma	Newly diagnosed	All patients	(Group CBT = Ind CBT)>NTC	1 year Group CBT> (Ind CBT=NTC); Coping skills & confusion
Moynihan et al. 1998	6 sessions APT	73	Testicular cancer	Newly diagnosed	All patients	CBT=NTC	1 year; Control>CBT
Moorey et al. 1998	8 sessions APT v. supportive counselling	47	Various cancers	All stages of disease	Patients referred to psycho-oncology service	CBT>ST	2 months CBT>ST

APT: adjuvant pschological therapy; CBT: cognitive behaviour therapy; ST: supportive therapy; NTC: no-treatment control.

90 minutes duration. One of five different instructional modes was presented each week:

- Relaxation and stress management.
- Communication and assertion.
- Problem solving and constructive thinking.
- Feelings management.
- Pleasant activity planning.

Participants rehearsed skills in the session through the use of structured exercises and then practised them as homework assignments. The support group by contrast was unstructured. The group leader acted as a facilitator, encouraging discussion of feelings and identifying underlying themes such as helplessness and loss of control.

Patients receiving supportive therapy showed little improvement, whereas the untreated group actually showed a deterioration in psychological adjustment. The coping skills group demonstrated significantly greater improvement than the other two conditions. These gains were in areas such as affect, satisfaction with work, social activities, physical appearance and sexual intimacy, communication, and coping with medical procedures. Patients kept a diary of their homework practice, and the records confirmed that most used the coping skills on a daily basis. The authors suggested that the support group may have been less effective because the patients were too heterogeneous and the intervention too brief for group cohesion to have developed. Although an excellent study in many respects, the lack of any follow-up beyond the end of therapy assessment is a serious flaw since there could have been a delayed effect on patients' functioning (as was found by Fawzy *et al.* 1993).

Over a period of twenty years, Cunningham and colleagues have been developing and systematically evaluating a psychoeducational group approach to coping with cancer. Their brief intervention consists of six weekly sessions of 2 hours length. The first hour of each session is didactic (learning a specific coping skill, relaxation, use of mental imagery, cognitive restructuring, goal definition, and problem solving) and the second hour is supportive (sharing of experiences and feelings). Participants are given a workbook and two tapes and encouraged to practise skills learned in the sessions as homework.

In their first controlled trial (Cunningham *et al.* 1989) with this approach this mixture of support and psychoeducational therapy was compared with six weeks of support alone. The patients were sixty consecutive referrals to the coping skills training programme. The sample was heterogeneous (various diagnoses, half with recurrent disease, half currently undergoing cancer treatment). Assessments were carried out at the start and end of therapy and 2–3 weeks after the end of therapy. Fifty-three patients completed the trial. Both groups showed significant improvements in psychological adjustment, but the psychoeducational group had a greater effect. A separate group of thirty-nine patients received the coping skills training and were not randomized—the improvements in mood were largely maintained at 3 months follow-up. These changes seem to be mediated by changes in perceived self-efficacy (Cunningham *et al.* 1991), are applicable to various cancer types and stages of disease, and can be delivered by therapists with different backgrounds (Cunningham *et al.* 1993).

Because of distance from the treatment centre or side-effects of treatment it often proves difficult for patients to attend six weekly sessions. The research team therefore devised an intensive weekend version of the programme. Both interventions produced statistically significant improvements which persisted at 3 month follow-up, even though the health of many of the participants deteriorated (Cunningham and Tocco 1995). Following the promising results of the study by Spiegel *et al.* (1989; see Chapter 4), which demonstrated an effect of long-term group therapy on survival of women with metastatic breast cancer, Cunningham and colleagues evaluated the effects of lengthening their programme (Edmonds *et al.* 1999). The longer term group intervention comprised 35 weekly 2 hour support groups, with a 20 week course of CBT assignments completed by patients at home and discussed in the group and a weekend intensive coping skills course. From 130 patients attending an intake inter-view, 66 were finally randomized into the study. Thirty received the intervention and 36 were in the control group. The control subjects received treatment as usual as well as the workbook and audiotapes used in the coping skills training. In the long-term intervention patients experienced more anxious preoccupation and less helplessness than the controls but no improvement in mood or quality of life. The authors report that there were profound clinical changes in the women attending the group, but these were not picked up by the conventional measures of psychosocial adjustment.

Another psychoeducational group approach which has been investigated inten-sively is that of Fawzy and colleagues (Fawzy and Fawzy 1994). Seven to ten patients meet for 90 minutes over a period of six weeks. The group contains four components:

- health education
- enhancement of illness-related problem-solving skills
- stress management (including relaxation)
- psychological support.

The treatment has been evaluated with patients with malignant melanoma. Eighty consecutive patients with stage I or II malignant melanoma (primary of local lymph node involvement) were randomly allocated to therapy or a no treatment control group. Two people were excluded from the analysis of the treatment group (one was a patient who died early in the intervention, the other was clinically depressed). Twelve were excluded from the control group (ten dropped out when informed they were assigned to the control group; there was incomplete data on two). Assessments were carried out at baseline, 6 weeks, and 6 months after intervention. At the end of therapy the only significant difference between the groups in adjustment was on the vigour scale of the Profile of Mood States (POMS) (McNair *et al.* 1971). At the 6 month follow-up, the intervention group showed significantly less depression-dejection, fatigue-inertia, confusion-bewilderment, and total mood disturbance on the POMS. At the end of therapy the intervention group reported more active-behavioural coping, and at 6 months more active-behavioural and active-cognitive coping than the control group. This brief treatment produced marked gains at follow-up, and also had an impact on survival (Fawzy *et al.* 1993; see Chapter 4). One methodological flaw in this study is the lack of an intention to treat design and the differential dropout from the two groups. In order to carry out a statistical analysis all the subjects must be randomized to a particular condition and included in the analysis. The fact that the 25 per cent of subjects who dropped out of the control condition did not differ in terms of age, sex, degree of disease, or other demographic variables, does not mean they were identical to those who participated. It is possible that these subjects had something of a fighting spirit and would have shown an improvement in psychological adjustment through their own coping strategies over the 6 month follow-up. This would mean that those left in the control group had a poorer psychological prognosis. Fawzy *et al.* (1996) have also compared individual with group treatment and found group treatment to be superior (see Chapter 13).

Mindfulness meditation is a development of meditation techniques used in Buddhism that has been shown to be useful in the treatment of anxiety disorders (Kabat-Zinn *et al.* 1992; Miller *et al.* 1995) and chronic pain (Kabat-Zinn *et al.* 1985). It involves learning to apply a detached awareness to moment to moment sensations and thoughts. Speca *et al.* (2000) randomly allocated 90 people with cancer to a 7 week group programme which taught mindfulness-based stress reduction or to a waiting list control. Patients in the treated group showed lower scores on the POMS for total mood disturbance, and subscales of depression, anxiety, anger, and confusion and higher scores in vigour. The improvement in this sample compared very favourably with other CBT studies that had used the POMS as an outcome measure (Cunningham and Tocco 1989; Fawzy *et al.* 1990a).

Cognitive behaviour therapy groups

Psychoeducational groups are highly structured and didactic. Three studies have investigated the effects of more flexible cognitive behavioural interventions in a group format. Two of these (Bottomley *et al.* 1996; Edelman *et al.* 1999a) specifically incorporated techniques from APT.

Evans and Connis (1995) compared cognitive behavioural group therapy with supportive therapy in depressed cancer patients receiving radiotherapy. Seventy-two depressed cancer patients were randomly assigned to one of three conditions— cognitive-behavioural treatment, social support, or a no-treatment control condition. The cognitive-behavioural and social support therapies resulted in less depression, hostility, and somatization compared to the no-treatment control. The social support intervention also resulted in fewer psychiatric symptoms and reduced maladaptive interpersonal sensitivity and anxiety. Both therapies also produced improvements in psychosocial function compared with no treatment, but the social support groups demonstrated more changes at 6 month follow-up.

Bottomley *et al.* (1996) reported a pilot study comparing CBT with a social support group in 31 newly diagnosed, psychologically distressed cancer patients. Fourteen of the patients declined to have therapy and so were allocated to a 'decliners' non-intervention group. Nine patients received CBT and eight social support. After an 8-week intervention both groups showed limited improvement in psychological states and coping styles. The coping styles of the CBT patients improved significantly over those of patients in the other two groups. At 3 month follow-up no significant differences were observed between the two intervention groups, possibly because two CBT patients had died.

Table 3.4 Randomized controlled trials of group cognitive behavioural therapies in cancer

Study	Interventions	n	Cancer type	Stage of disease	Selection	Outcome	Follow-up
Heinrich & Schag 1985	6 sessions stress and activity management v. current available care	51	Commonly occurring cancers	Various stages	All patients	CBT=NTC; Both groups improved in psychosocial adjustment	2 months—CBT > NTC on coping in medical situations and achieving activity goals
Telch & Telch 1986	6 sessions group coping skills instruction v. supportive group therapy	41	Various cancers	Various stages of disease; Karnovsky > 70	Psychosocial distress	CBT > ST > NTC; NTC group deteriorated	None
Cunningham et al. 1989	6 sessions group psycho-educational therapy v. supportive discussion	53	Various cancers and stages of disease	Various stages of disease	Patients referred	CBT > ST	None
Fawzy et al. 1990; 1993	6 sessions group CBT v. standard medical treatment	68	Malignant melanoma	Newly diagnosed	All patients	CBT > NTC	6 months CBT > NTC
Evans et al. 1995	Group CBT v. social support v. no-treatment control	72			Depressed patients undergoing chemotherapy	(CBT = ST) > NTC Depression, hostility & somatisation; ST > NTC; Psychiatric symptoms	6 months ST > CBT > NTC

Study	Intervention	N	Cancer	Stage	Patients	Result	Follow-up
Bottomley et al. 1996	8 sessions group CBT v. support group v. non-intervention	31			Psychologically distressed patients	CBT = ST	3 months CBT = ST
Edelman et al. 1999	8 sessions group CBT v. treatment as usual	124	Breast cancer	Metastatic disease		CBT > NTC; Total mood & self esteem	3 & 6 months CBT = NTC
Edelman et al. 1999	12 sessions group CBT v. supportive therapy	60	Breast cancer	Newly diagnosed primary disease	All patients	CBT > ST; Quality of life and self-esteem	4 months CBT = ST
Edmonds et al. 1999	35 sessions group support, CBT + W/E course v. standard hospital care	66	Breast cancer	Metastatic disease	All patients	CBT + support = NTC	CBT + support = NTC
Speca et al. 2000	7 sessions mindfulness meditation-based stress reduction v. waiting list control	90	Various cancers	Various stages	All patients	CBT > NTC	None

CBT: cognitive behaviour therapy; ST: supportive therapy; NTC: no-treatment control.

Edelman *et al.* (1999b) compared CBT and supportive therapy in women with primary breast cancer. Sixty women were randomly allocated to either twelve sessions of group cognitive behaviour therapy or a supportive group therapy. Both groups showed improvements in depression, quality of life and self-esteem. There was significantly more improvement in quality of life and self-esteem in the CBT group compared to the supportive therapy group. The benefits of the CBT group over support were no longer present at 4 month follow-up.

Meta-analyses

Many of the studies described so far have suffered from the methodological drawback of small sample sizes. Meta-analysis is a statistical technique which attempts to overcome this problem by combining the results from several studies. Outcome measures are converted to a common measure (the effect size) so that individual effect sizes can be pooled. The effect size is calculated from the formula

$$\text{Effect size} = \frac{M_1 - M_2}{SD}$$

Where M_1 is the mean of the treatment group, M_2 the mean of the control group and SD the pooled standard deviation for the two groups. Meyer and Mark (1995) examined 45 trials of different psychological therapies in cancer patients, finding a small mean effect size of 0.24. Sheard and Maguire (1999) criticized this study on the basis that it had included too broad a selection of trials in terms of the research questions asked and the outcome measures used. They instead chose trials that had sought to treat either anxiety and/ or depression. Altogether 19 trials had included measures for anxiety. The overall effect size was 0.42 comparing treated patients and untreated controls. When the ten trials with the most reliable design were examined, the effect size was 0.36. Twenty trials had data on outcome of depression. The effect size for treated patients compared to untreated controls was 0.36. There was no difference between studies which used group therapies or individual therapies. Sheard and Maguire then went on to analyse studies that had selected patients on the basis of their experiencing or being at risk of psychological distress. In these studies the impact of therapy was much more substantial. Four trials in this category were associated with powerful effects. (Linn *et al.* 1982, Worden and Weisman 1984, Telch and Telch 1986, Greer *et al.* 1992). The effect sizes were 0.94 for anxiety and 0.85 for depression. These large effect sizes indicated that the average patient in the treatment conditions did better than 80% of patients in the untreated control conditions. Although the meta-analysis includes all forms of therapy, these four trials were all cognitive behavioural interventions.

This meta-analysis also revealed that group therapy was as effective as individual therapy, particularly in regard to psycho-educational courses, and that short but intensive interventions by highly trained therapists were more effective than protracted ones delivered by less psychologically trained staff.

The authors concluded that: 'preventative psychological interventions in cancer patients may have a moderate clinical effect upon anxiety but not depression. There are indications that interventions targeted at those at risk or suffering significant psychological distress have strong clinical effects. Evidence on the effectiveness of such targeted interventions and of the feasibility and effects of group therapy in a European context is required.'

Conclusions

Despite the heterogeneity of these studies some common themes are beginning to emerge from the literature. Most of the studies confirm the effectiveness of cognitive behavioural interventions compared to 'treatment as usual' conditions. This is particularly clear from the studies which have taken patients who are psychologically distressed. All trials have demonstrated the superiority of CBT over no treatment for distressed individuals (Telch and Telch 1986; Evans and Connis 1995; Greer *et al.* 1992; Moorey *et al.* 1998). These differences have been shown to persist for at least a year (Moorey *et al.* 1994). Most of the trials have demonstrated a superiority of CBT over 'treatment as usual' when all patients are entered into the trial, but the effect size of this intervention is small compared to that with psychologically distressed patients. The cost-effectiveness of intervention with unselected patients can be questioned. Structured psychoeducational programmes are probably the intervention of choice with non-distressed patients.

The advantage of CBT over other psychological treatments is not firmly established. The comparison treatment is usually some form of supportive/non-directive therapy. Four trials have shown CBT to be more effective at the end of therapy (Telch and Telch 1986; Cunningham and Tocco 1989; Edelman *et al.* 1999b; Moorey *et al.* 1998) and three have shown the therapies to be equally effective (Evans and Connis 1995; Bottomley *et al.* 1996; Edmonds *et al.* 1999).

Most studies have used heterogeneous groups of patients, so it is not yet possible to make judgements about which types of cancer CBT may or may not work with. Definite evidence exists for efficacy with breast cancer (Edelman *et al.* 1999a, b) and malignant melanoma (Fawzy *et al.* 1990a, 1996). The single study with testicular cancer failed to find an effect (Moynihan *et al.* 1998). There is no evidence to suggest that people with metastatic or more advanced disease do less well with CBT than people with early cancer.

There is evidence that intervening too early may not be beneficial to cancer patients. Moynihan *et al.* (1998) found that many of their men with testicular cancer did not wish to receive counselling, and that those who did received little benefit. The trend for the control group to do better at a year raises the possibility that intervening too early may be detrimental! Edgar's finding (Edgar *et al.* 1992) that waiting for seven months before intervening produced better results than intervening in the first three months confirms the view that routine early intervention is not indicated. It may be that giving therapy too soon in some way interferes with the natural coping process, perhaps robbing people of their sense of personal control over their emotional recovery from the shock of cancer. We do not yet know if this applies only to CBT (in which case it might be that too problem-focused a treatment early on interferes with emotional processing) or whether it applies to all forms of psychological therapy.

The evidence from studies of post traumatic stress disorder that critical incident debriefing may be harmful suggests that this could be the case for any form of psychological intervention given too early (Wessely *et al.* 2000).

We can therefore affirm that CBT, whether given in group or individual form, does indeed improve the quality of life of people with cancer, and that it is certainly as effective as supportive therapy or perhaps more effective. Further work is needed to establish which patients benefit most from which type of treatment. More studies of people with advanced disease and terminal illness are needed. Targeting distressed patients, rather than trying to treat all patients, is the most efficient way of using the limited resources of cognitive behaviour therapists.

Chapter 4

Can psychological therapy affect duration of survival?

In an astonishing clinical report published in 1848, John Elliotson, a British physician, claimed that he had successfully treated a woman with cancer of the right breast ('scirrhus cancer') by means of hypnosis conducted for five years. During that period, the tumour shrank and then disappeared completely. Elliotson's (1848) report is of historical interest only. The vast majority of the medical profession, including the present authors, have always assumed that the course of cancer cannot be influenced by any psychological intervention. This assumption, however, was challenged in 1989 by Spiegel and his colleagues in their landmark study of women with metastatic breast cancer. Their randomized clinical trial revealed that patients who received group therapy ($n=50$) survived for an average of 18.9 months longer than patients in the control group ($n=36$) who did not receive group therapy (Spiegel *et al.* 1989).

'Supportive/expressive' group therapy was conducted weekly for at least one year. According to Spiegel (1985) this therapy comprised four components:

1 Patients were encouraged to express their feelings and fears concerning their illness. They encouraged each other to be assertive and to recognize and express anger in appropriate ways. Anxiety about death and dying was addressed directly.

2 Physical symptoms were addressed, for example by teaching the women how to control their experience of pain by means of self-hypnosis and relaxation.

3 Mutual support figured prominently during therapy.

4 Issues concerning meaning of life were explored; patients reassessed their life values, focusing on projects that were still possible during the remainder of their lives. Spiegel observed that the sense of extracting meaning from tragedy was an important aspect of therapy.

It is not surprising that Spiegel's study created enormous interest. For the first time, a randomized controlled investigation had demonstrated that psychological intervention—in this case, supportive/expressive group therapy for one year—had a significant, favourable effect on the survival of patients with metastatic cancer. This finding was completely unexpected since the study had been designed to determine the effect of group therapy on mood disturbance (Classen *et al.* 1998). Spiegel and his colleagues looked for other possible explanations for their finding by testing 26 variables, including age, initial staging, number of days of irradiation, type of surgery, interval from first diagnosis to death, degree of metastatic spread, for baseline differences between the therapy and control groups that could account for the survival difference. None of these variables explained the difference in duration of survival. Having exhausted other possibilities, the authors drew the logical conclusion that the difference in survival time was due to group therapy. Strenuous efforts have been made to refute this conclusion by Fox (1998a). He argued that the survival curve for patients in the control group looked unusually steep. When compared with that of a population with metastatic cancer from the same region, the control patients surviving longer than 20 months were 'an extremely aberrant sample subject to the strong biasing influence of possible confounders, of which a considerable number are known but not including those accounted for in the study'. His criticisms were answered in detail by Spiegel *et al.* (1998); this was followed by a rejoinder from Fox (1998b) which, in turn, produced strong arguments against Fox's views from Goodwin *et al.* (1999) and Speca (1999) followed by yet another rejoinder by Fox (1999). The debate highlights the formidable problems in this particular area of research. Readers with an interest in methodology will find the debate informative. In our view, Spiegel and his colleagues' study meets the customary requirements of scientific evidence. But, as Spiegel himself points out, replication studies are necessary before any general conclusions can be made.

Since Spiegel's study, several other investigations have been reported though none are replication studies. Richardson and colleagues (1990) studied 94 patients with various haematological cancers. Patients were randomly assigned to one of three treatment conditions or to a control group. The treatment conditions comprised either an educational programme and a home visit, or the same educational programme plus 'shaping' or education plus 'shaping' plus a home visit. The education programme was carried out by a trained nurse who described in detail the disease and its treatment, emphasizing the importance of compliance with treatment and persuading family members to ensure that the patient took the prescribed drugs. 'Shaping' involved the nurse working with the patient so that the latter learnt to take responsibility for self-medication. At follow-up 2 to 5 years later, patients in all the educational intervention groups had an improved survival rate compared with patients in the control group. This finding held good after differences in treatment compliance were taken into account.

Of particular interest is the investigation of 68 patients with stage I and II malignant melanoma carried out by Fawzy and his colleagues (1990b, 1993). Their psychological intervention consisted of six weekly sessions of group therapy which were focused on health education, stress management, coping skills, and group support. Patients were randomly allocated to the support group or a control group. Their outcome measures included immune responses and psychological responses up to 6 months after the psychological intervention and survival 5 to 6 years later. With regard to immune responses, psychological intervention was associated with a significant increase in the percentage of natural killer cells, in natural killer cell activity, and in CD8 (suppressor/cytotoxic) T cells. Higher levels of natural killer cell activity predicted survival. Psychological intervention significantly reduced depression, fatigue and mood disturbance, and enhanced coping skills. At 6-year follow-up, patients in the control group had a significantly higher death rate (10 out of 34) than patients who had received psychological intervention (3 out of 24). Fawzy and Fawzy (1994) concluded that: 'psychiatric interventions that enhance effective coping and reduce affective distress appear to have beneficial effects on survival'.

Each of the studies considered so far has reported significant associations between duration of survival and either group therapy (Spiegel *et al.* 1989; Fawzy *et al.* 1990, 1993) or an educational programme (Richardson *et al.* 1990). There are, however, other psychological intervention studies which have not found any effect on survival. In the first of these studies, Linn *et al.* (1982) examined the effect of individual supportive psychotherapy on 120 men with various metastatic cancers (predominantly lung cancer). Therapy focused on encouraging patients to express their feelings, to exert personal control—where possible—in their lives, and to find some meaning in their lives. Patients were randomly allocated to a therapy group and a control group. At follow-up 1 year later, duration of survival was similar in both groups. A second study with negative results was reported by Ilnyckyj *et al.* (1994). A series of 127 patients with a variety of cancers at various disease stages was studied. Patients were randomly assigned to a control group or to one of three psychological intervention groups. Psychological therapy consisted of weekly sessions of 'group therapy' for six months. One group was led by a social worker, another group was led by a social worker for three months and then 'peer-led', whereas the third group was entirely 'peer-led'. It is not clear what kind of group therapy was given. At follow-up eleven years later, duration of survival was found to be similar among patients in the control and therapy groups. This study suffers from lack of information concerning the nature of the psychological interventions.

Another investigation to be considered here is a randomized controlled trial of group therapy by Cunningham and his colleagues (1998). They studied women with metastatic breast cancer, 30 of whom received 35 weekly sessions of supportive plus cognitive behavioural therapy. The control group consisted of 36 women who received only a home study cognitive behavioural package. At 5-year follow-up, the authors found no significant difference in survival between the therapy and control groups. However, the numbers were small and may have been insufficient to reveal survival difference. Furthermore, the control group was not a no-treatment group; patients in the control group made use of relaxation audio tapes and 28% attended an outside support group. There is, therefore, some doubt about these negative results. The authors themselves state: 'yet our clinical impression, in agreement with that of many who have long experience of psychological work with cancer patients … is that some patients, particularly those who become very involved in trying to help themselves, do much better than is expected medically'.

A recent study of group cognitive behaviour therapy (CBT) for patients with metastatic breast cancer was carried out by Edelman and her colleagues (1999a). One hundred and twenty-four patients were randomly allocated to CBT or a standard care control group. Three patients were subsequently found not to have metastatic disease and were therefore excluded. Data regarding known medical prognostic factors were obtained. CBT comprised a core programme of eight weekly sessions and a 'family night' followed by three further monthly sessions. Patients were taught a range of cognitive and behavioural strategies such as thought monitoring, cognitive restructuring, goal setting, and homework excercises. Statistical analysis of 121 patients entered in the study at 2 to 5 year follow-up revealed no survival advantage associated with CBT.

Is randomization appropriate?

Cunningham et al. (1998) have put forward an interesting suggestion. In their experience, relatively few patients make the kind of substantial psychological changes (in lifestyle, attitudes, awareness of mind–body connections and other factors) which could influence their physiology sufficiently to affect duration of survival. Such highly motivated people tend not to be common or available for randomized group assignment. They are individuals who take steps to get the therapy they want. Hence, if only a small proportion of the patients undergoing psychological intervention make significant changes, the effects may be lost when group medians are calculated and compared, unless the number of subjects is very large. In addition, the distribution of such highly motivated patients in small experimental groups may be greatly influenced by chance. Cunningham argues that, instead of randomization, a different kind of experimental design is more appropriate, namely single case studies in which individuals are followed up for years and changes in their psychological functioning are compared with the extent to which these patients outlive their predicted survival according to medical prognostic features.

These are persuasive arguments. There may well be a place for single case studies in which the patient is his or her own control (Aldridge 1992). However, a serious weakness of single case studies is that unlike randomized studies, one cannot make valid generalizations. Admittedly, randomized controlled trials have certain limitations. Ethical problems arise in deciding whether and when it is justified to compare a new treatment with current treatment or with no active treatment. There are often considerable difficulties in explaining randomization to patients and obtaining genuine informed consent. Large numbers of patients are required in order to ensure—as far as possible—that the experimental and control groups are similar in all respects other than the treatment under investigation. Moreover, results of randomized trials are based on comparisons between group means and do not tell us whether any given individual patient will benefit from psychological intervention. As one critic puts it, 'randomization tends to obscure rather than illuminate interactive effects between treatments and personal characteristics' (Weinstein 1974). On the other hand, there can be no doubt that prospective controlled trials are essential if we are to avoid or minimize the influence of bias. Randomization is not the only way to attempt to avoid bias—matching is another—but randomizing to experimental and control groups is regarded by most investigators as the most effective and bias-free methodology (Bradford Hill 1961; Cawley 1983; Fox 1998a; Spiegel et al. 1998). For this reason, we have considered only randomized controlled studies in this review. Randomization, as we have noted, has its problems. But in the absence of a demonstrably superior method of eliminating bias we are stuck with it. Winston Churchill once described democracy as the least worst form of government; similarly, randomization could be regarded as the least worst method of dealing with bias.

Conclusions

Only seven randomized controlled studies have been reported so far. These studies reveal conflicting results regarding the influence of psychological intervention on duration of survival among patients with cancer. These inconsistent findings are not surprising given that the cited studies are based on small numbers of patients with different types and stages of cancer undergoing different kinds of psychological intervention. Since the studies are not comparable, no definitive conclusions can be drawn. Clearly careful rigorous replication studies are required. Fortunately, two such replication studies of Spiegel's original study are in progress (Classen *et al.* 1996; Goodwin *et al.* 1996). The results of these studies are awaited with great interest.

PART TWO

Cognitive Behaviour Therapy

Chapter 5

Overview of therapy

The place of psychological treatment in oncology

Since the first edition of this book, the field of psychosocial oncology has grown considerably. Although by no means widespread, psychological support and treatment is available in many oncology services. The form this help takes and the training and expertise of those who give it varies considerably. In many units oncology nurses may have some training in counselling skills. Some services are fortunate in having specialist nurses working with breast cancer or in palliative care whose main role is attending to the psychosocial needs of cancer patients. Less frequently, liaison psychiatrists may have attachments to cancer units, and clinical psychologists may also be on hand to deliver cognitive behavioural and other treatments. There is no consensus about how psychosocial services in oncology should best be organized. Providing for the psychological and social needs of people with cancer can be considered under three broad headings:

Development of skills among health professionals

Nurses and doctors working in oncology should all possess basic skills in communication skills (Faulkner *et al.* 1991; Parle *et al.* 1997) including breaking bad news (Girgis and Sanson-Fisher 1998), identifying and managing distress, providing information, and recognizing problems that require intervention from a more specialist service.

Provision of interventions within oncology services

Staff working within oncology departments may have specific skills in counselling or other psychological interventions. These interventions may take the form of brief informal therapy or longer term support as part of the work of nurse specialists or social workers. They may also take the form of groups such as relaxation groups, psychoeducational groups, and support groups. Patients themselves may be able to help in these settings by sharing their own experiences of what cancer has meant to them and how they have coped.

Specialist psycho-oncology services

More complicated adjustment reactions, and moderate to severe anxiety and depression will often need more specialist help, usually from clinical psychologists, liaison nurses, or liaison psychiatrists. Access to a psychiatrist is particularly important when questions about the management of psychological syndromes which might have an organic origin or issues of assessment of suicide risk arise. For these arrangements to work well, the mental health professional is best seen as an integral member of the oncology team so that the patient and family's emotional and interpersonal needs are given as much weight as purely medical considerations.

It was for this reason that we chose the name 'adjuvant psychological therapy' (APT) for our particular brand of cognitive behaviour therapy. Just as one might expect to receive adjuvant chemotherapy, it should be equally acceptable to receive adjuvant psychological therapy (Cunningham 1995). APT is designed to be used alongside and as an aid to physical forms of treatment in an integrated treatment setting. With its emphasis on fostering a positive attitude, helping the patient to collaborate with and cope with treatment, and reducing emotional distress, this form of therapy can complement traditional medical treatment. Some of the theoretical and clinical components of APT can be used in all three areas of psychosocial oncology. For instance, when a patient is considering whether or not to go ahead with a course of chemotherapy an oncologist could collaboratively help the patient to assess the costs and benefits of the treatment (see Chapter 9). Cognitive behavioural techniques can be used more formally by specialist breast-care nurses or MacMillan nurses either in group or individual format. Clinical psychologists and psychiatrists will find this therapy particularly applicable to the more distressed patients referred to them.

APT is intended for use across a broad spectrum of problems extending from people with no abnormal symptoms who want help in fighting and coping with cancer, to those with definable psychiatric illness. However, most patients will access this therapy because they are having difficulties in coping. People undergoing adjustment reactions constitute the largest group referred for psychological treatment. With these patients more emphasis may be placed on non-directive techniques in the first instance, facilitating expression of negative emotions before moving on to the problem-solving components of therapy. With mild to moderate depression or anxiety APT looks very much like a standard cognitive behaviour therapy. Ventilation may be less important, particularly if there is a well-established, chronic maladaptive adjustment style. Couples problems and sexual problems associated with cancer can also be addressed with this approach, but in relationships with long-standing conflict or disturbance the impact of cancer is often of secondary importance. A brief-focused therapy such as APT which is aimed primarily at improving personal and marital adjustment to physical disease may be unsuitable, and these couples may need formal marital or family therapy. There are well-established cognitive behaviour approaches to these problems which can be applied to people with cancer (Beck 1988; Dattilio and Padesky 1990; Dattilio 1997).

Anticipatory nausea occurs in up to 15% of patients treated with chemotherapy. Nausea and anxiety are experienced shortly before receiving chemotherapy, and may be triggered by specific environmental cues such as syringes, white coats, or hospitals. This condition responds very well to a combination of cognitive and behavioural treatments (Watson and Marvell 1992; Watson 1993) and these treatment methods can be used by health professionals without extensive psychological therapy training (Morrow *et al.* 1992).

Cancer pain can also be alleviated to some degree with cognitive behavioural techniques (Turk and Fernandez 1991).

APT is not suitable for people who are actively psychotic. The cognitive behavioural techniques that have been applied successfully in schizophrenia (Kingdon and Turkington 1994; Kuipers *et al.* 1997) require special training and experience. This does not mean that people with a diagnosis of schizophrenia who are in remission, or whose psychotic symptoms are reasonably well controlled cannot benefit from APT. The same proviso applies to people with organic psychoses such as confusional states or dementia. It is important to work closely with the oncologists treating the patient to ensure that any organic causes of psychological reactions have been investigated and treated before embarking on a course of APT. People with more severe forms of depression or anxiety states will often require a combination of psychotherapy and pharmacological treatment. Tarrier and Maguire (1984) found that a brief cognitive behavioural treatment of four sessions' duration was more effective for depressed patients with breast cancer when given in combination with antidepressant medication.

Most patients with adjustment reactions can be treated with APT in the form described in this book. Table 5.1 summarizes the forms of psychological disturbance encountered in oncology and gives guidelines for the use of APT with each condition.

The theoretical basis of APT

The cognitive model of adjustment (see Chapter 2) proposes that it is the appraisals, interpretations, and evaluations that the individual makes about cancer that determine his or her emotional and behavioural reactions. It is not the symptoms of the disease or the effects of treatment *per se* which produce the emotional response, but the meanings they hold for the person involved. How he or she thinks about the illness and its implications for his or her life is central to adjustment. If the predominant meaning of cancer is loss, the person will feel depressed. If cancer represents a potential threat to health, security, or life itself, the emotional response will be one of anxiety. However, if the person sees the disease as an intrusion and unjust violation of his or her world the reaction will be one of anger. Adjustment involves an interpretation of the type of stress cancer imposes, evaluation of how well the stress can be managed and the mobilization of coping behaviours. Emotional reactions will vary as the disease itself changes or the person seeks different ways to interpret his or her situation.

Table 5.1 Psychological disturbances encountered in oncology and guidelines for the application of APT

Suitability for APT	Disorder
Suitable	Adjustment reactions; Depression; Anxiety; Sexual problems; Couples problems; Anticipatory nausea; Pain
	Possibly suitable (may require modified treatment, e.g. combination with drug therapy, or longer duration of treatment) Severe depression; Severe anxiety; Co-existing personality disorder; Alcohol abuse; Major pre-existing couples problems
Unsuitable	Active psychoses; Schizophrenia; Bipolar affective disorder; Organic psychoses; Confusional states; Dementia

Everyone has a set of basic assumptions about themselves and their world (as shown in Chapter 2), which do not usually include beliefs that they will develop cancer. One of the tasks for the individual with cancer is to make sense of the diagnosis, either by incorporating the experience into their world-view, or modifying their beliefs. Some authorities insist that cancer makes people modify their beliefs by realizing the world is not benevolent (Janoff-Bulman 1999). Others point to the way an individual can manage to retain 'positive illusions', for instance by stressing that there are other people who are worse off, even in the face of serious illness (Taylor *et al.* 2000).

After an initial period of turmoil most patients develop a relatively stable adjustment style. The most significant threat that cancer poses is to the very survival of the patient. There are five common adjustment styles, as described in Chapter 2 (fighting spirit; denial; fatalism; helplessness and hopelessness; anxious preoccupation), and each represents a slightly different way of viewing the threat to survival. These form a constellation of thoughts, feelings and behaviours which the individual uses to cope. The individual adjustment style can be seen as a cognitive schema. It is like a template which makes sense of the disease, its treatment, the individual's response, and the outcome in the future. People with maladaptive adjustment styles tend to have a rigid schema. There is a cognitive triad which involves a negative view of the diagnosis, control of the disease, and its prognosis. For instance, the patient with a helpless/hopeless response sees the diagnosis as a death sentence, believes there is nothing anyone can do about it, and feels hopeless about the future. Information about cancer is processed in a biased fashion. Cognitive distortions maintain the helpless/hopeless schema by filtering out hopeful information while magnifying negative information about the disease. Patients will overgeneralize from a single event: 'I felt too ill to do much today; I'll never be able to do the things I want to do.' Or they may think in a black and white fashion: 'If I can't do everything I used to do, there's no point in doing anything.' The more entrenched the maladaptive adjustment style, the more negative is the thinking. These patients have frequent *negative automatic thoughts* which may be very unrealistic and exaggerated. These negative thoughts maintain the patient's emotional distress, and prevent effective coping strategies being used. Other modes of adjustment operate in a similar way. There is obviously a spectrum ranging from realistic to unrealistic thoughts and attitudes about the disease, and for many people with advanced disease a pessimistic view of their prognosis is correct, but maladaptive adjustment styles distort reality to make it even bleaker than it really is. The helpless/hopeless patient with advanced disease will focus on his or her inability to do anything about the disease or quality of life, instead of looking at ways in which the disease can be controlled and the quality of life which is left enhanced.

The meaning of cancer and the threat of death are probably the most important factors influencing patients' adjustment. For some people other factors related to the disease may be of more significance. There may be a realistic belief about the possibility of recovery, but the side-effects of treatment may seem intolerable.

Some patients are distressed by the effects of surgery and if the emotional upset experienced is severe or prolonged it will require help. There are often negative automatic thoughts which reflect unrealistic self-deprecation. Patients may think: I'm hideous, 'I can't go out like this'; 'No one could possibly love me'. For others it may be

Table 5.2 Patients' perceptions of diagnosis, degree of personal control and prognosis in different adjustment styles

	Survival schema		
Adjustment style	**Diagnosis**	**Control**	**Prognosis**
Fighting spirit	Challenge	Person believes he can control the disease and/or life	Good
Denial	Minimal threat	Irrelevant	Good
Fatalism	Minimal or major threat	Believes others can control the situation but the person cannot	Unknown
Helpless/ hopeless	Major threat, loss or defeat	Believes nothing can affect disease outcome	Poor
Anxious preoccupation	Major threat	Person uncertain about their ability to exert control over disease	Uncertain

the effects of the disease on significant areas of their lives which cause problems. Many men consider themselves less worthwhile if they have to give up employment as a result of cancer. These factors usually imply some sort of threat to the person's self-image through loss of attractiveness, role, or self-esteem etc. Prior to cancer an individual has a fairly stable view of him- or herself in relation to other people and the world. This can be seen as a self schema which integrates memories, beliefs, and goals related to the self-image. Cancer does not necessarily impinge upon this. But in some cases the effects of cancer or its treatment may become a serious threat to the self. For instance, if people have a strong belief that they can only be happy if others find them attractive, any disfigurement as a result of treatment can seriously damage their self-esteem. Patients who have difficulty in coping may develop a negative image of themselves as ugly, diseased, or unlovable. Patients who experience a threat to their usual self-image will experience intense anxiety, for example if a woman believes that chemotherapy will make her bald and unattractive. These two areas of threat, to *survival* and to the *self*, may exist separately or together and the cognitive structures involved interact.

If this survival schema becomes more generalized it can apply to areas of the patient's life which are unrelated to cancer. A helpless/hopeless response can turn into depression as negative thinking becomes generalized to views about the self, the world, and the future unrelated to the disease. An anxious preoccupation can generalize to become an anxiety state. In coming to a stable adjustment style, patients often go through many different interpretations of their situation. Feelings of anger, sadness and fear are a normal part of this adjustment process. It may be that a certain degree of emotional processing is necessary to develop an adaptive way of coping with the disease. Patients who avoid these emotions, or who do not have a supportive social network in which to express them, may encounter difficulties in adapting to the disease.

The final component of the theory behind APT concerns the interactive nature of coping with cancer. The disease occurs in a social context, and important people in the patient's life will influence his or her feelings. Friends, relatives and health professionals will all give informational and emotional support. The interpretation the patient places on the behaviour of these people will contribute to the emotional response observed. A woman with breast cancer believed that the reactions of her friends to news of her illness would be a mixture of pity and gossip so she determined to tell no one of her diagnosis. Another woman with ovarian cancer discovered that by telling people of her diagnosis she felt a sense of relief and also a feeling of self-confidence that she could reveal this, even if her friends' reactions were less support-ive than she had hoped.

The partner plays a very important role in the patient's coping. The dynamics of the marital relationship can often be dramatically affected by cancer. Suppression of emo-tions, particularly anger, can lead to communication problems between the patient and the partner which require psychological help.

From this theoretical framework it is possible to generate the aims of therapy:

Aims of adjuvant psychological therapy

1 To reduce emotional distress.
2 To improve mental adjustment to cancer by inducing a positive fighting spirit.
3 To promote in patients a sense of personal control over their lives and active participation in the treatment of their cancer.
4 To develop effective coping strategies for dealing with cancer-related problems.
5 To improve communication between the patient and partner.
6 To encourage open expression of feelings, particularly anger and other negative feelings in a safe environment.

Format of therapy

APT developed as a modification of Beck's cognitive therapy. Experience in treating people with cancer at King's College Hospital and The Royal Marsden Hospital, London generated a number of practical strategies for dealing with the problems of this group of patients. This clinical experience has been used to adapt the cognitive therapy methods traditionally employed with patients suffering from states of anxiety and depression. APT is carried out over 6–12 weekly sessions of an hour's duration. Therapy is problem-oriented: problems encountered may be emotional (e.g. depres-sion), interpersonal (e.g. problems in communicating with the partner), or related to the cancer type (e.g. body image problems of mastectomy patients). The patient is taught the cognitive model of adjustment to cancer and shown how his or her thoughts contribute to distress. This educational component is important since it provides the rationale for the coping strategies the patient learns during therapy. Each therapy session is structured by setting an agenda to deal with one or more of these problems. Regular homework assignments are used to give the patient experience of finding alternative, more constructive ways of thinking and developing new coping strategies.

The therapeutic relationship is one of 'collaborative empiricism': the patient is taught to examine his or her beliefs about cancer, and to treat them as hypotheses that can be tested. If someone has early stage disease with a good prognosis, a statement such as: 'I know I'll be dead by next year' is tested by considering the evidence for and against it. Often beliefs are based upon misconceptions or no evidence at all. Even when cancer is more advanced such a thought may be overly pessimistic, because it assumes an inevitable certainty about the course of the disease. The therapist also collaborates with the patient to find and employ strategies for coping with cancer. Therapy is conceptualized as a joint problem-solving exercise, where the insights and suggestions of the patient and partner can be as useful as those of the therapist.

Components of APT

Emotional expression

Although emotional expression is unlikely to be therapeutic if it is the sole procedure in a therapy, it can have an important place as part of treatment for patients undergoing adjustment reactions. Ventilation of feelings is often needed before a problem-solving approach can be used. Anger seems to be one emotion which people with cancer find hard to express (Watson *et al.* 1984), and APT therefore sets out to facilitate the constructive expression of anger (see Chapter 7).

Behavioural techniques

Behavioural techniques are usually employed in the early stages of therapy. Techniques are the same as those used in cognitive behavioural therapies for anxiety and depression, including graded task assignments and activity scheduling, behavioural experiments, relaxation, and distraction. Cancer robs patients of control of their own bodies, and its treatment involves more passivity than the treatment of other conditions. This loss of control can spread to other areas of patients' lives. Behavioural techniques help to give a sense of mastery or control over the patient's life and environment. Behavioural assignments can help the person develop a sense of control over the disease itself through encouraging co-operation with treatment or self-help techniques like visualization. They can also develop control in areas unrelated to cancer and indirectly foster a fighting spirit.

Cognitive techniques

During the session the therapist elicits automatic thoughts associated with the problems the patient is facing and shows the person how to identify his or her own negative thoughts. From the first or second session the patient is set the task of monitoring thoughts between sessions. Once these cognitions can be recognized, the next step is to learn to test them. A variety of techniques can be used for this process of cognitive restructuring. *Reality-testing* involves examining the evidence for a particular thought or belief. This allows realistic, sad or anxious thoughts to be distinguished from distorted negative thinking. A technique which can be used with distressing realistic thoughts as well as unrealistic ones is the *search for alternatives*. The patient is encouraged to explore all the possible explanations, predictions, or ways of looking at something to see if more realistic or more positive alternatives are available. *Decatastrophizing* encourages the patient to think about what he or she fears to see if it is really that bad. For instance, a patient who is terrified of recurrence can consider what treatment might be available and what methods of fighting the disease he or she might develop if it did recur. Testing the *effect of negative thinking* helps to show that even when a thought is realistic it is not necessarily helpful, because it may interfere with the person's ability to problem solve or get on with their life. When the patient can recognize these negative automatic thoughts, more realistic or more constructive thoughts are used as responses. Often the cognitive change will suggest a *behavioural plan* that can help to consolidate the new way of thinking. If the person is less convinced that the alternative way of thinking is that appropriate, they can try *behavioural experiments* to test the old and new beliefs.

Working with couples

Partners are involved in two main ways in APT. They can act as powerful co-therapists, reminding patients of their strengths, remembering times when they have coped effectively in the past and providing reinforcement for successful coping efforts. Couples problems are addressed using a combination of cognitive and behavioural techniques with a strong emphasis on facilitating communication.

Characteristics of APT

The following chapters in this section will describe the techniques in more detail. Because it uses behavioural, cognitive, emotion-focused, and interpersonal techniques, APT can be called a multimodal therapy (see Box 1). The techniques are

Box 1 Characteristics of APT—based on a cognitive model of adjustment to cancer

- structured
- short-term (6–12 sessions)
- focused and problem-oriented
- educational (patient is taught coping strategies)
- collaborative
- makes use of homework assignments
- uses a variety of treatment techniques: non-directive methods; behavioural techniques; cognitive techniques; interpersonal techniques.

tailored to the particular needs of the individual. Some people do not have partners and so individual therapy is the only method available. Some people need to spend a lot of time just talking about their feelings; others can move into a problem-solving mode straight away. Many patients make rapid gains with behavioural techniques alone and do not take to cognitive techniques, whereas others do not show any behavioural deficits and so cognitive interventions are the main therapeutic method.

Phases of therapy

This flexible approach means that aims and techniques are changed and developed over the course of therapy in response to the patient's needs. It is not possible to lay down hard and fast rules about the course of therapy. However, it is sometimes useful to consider the treatment as three broad phases. These phases usually have slightly different aims, and different techniques are emphasized as a result.

Beginning therapy

The aims of the initial stage of therapy are:

1. *Symptom relief:* the therapist works with the patient to develop coping strategies for immediate problems. These will usually be either emotional distress, such as depression and anxiety, or life crises. Problem-solving and behavioural techniques such as distraction, relaxation, graded task assignment and activity scheduling are used in this phase.

2. *Living an ordinary life:* the therapist explains the principles of maximizing the quality of life available. Patient and partner are helped to plan as active and rewarding a time together as is possible within the constraints of the disease. The daily activity schedule is used as a basis for this. Activity scheduling helps to:

build on strengths;

use mastery and pleasure experiences to promote control; and

encourage patient and partner to plan new goals.

3. *Teaching the cognitive model:* aims (1) and (2) above should be met within a cognitive framework. As problems are defined and addressed they are formulated in cognitive terms. The therapist repeatedly uses examples from the person's thoughts and feelings. It may be possible with some people to begin thought monitoring during this stage.

4. *Encouraging open expression of feelings:* the person is encouraged to express and accept negative emotions such as anger and despair before they are subjected to any reality testing. The art of APT lies in getting the right balance between facing the fears of cancer and positively avoiding them through the active approach described in (2) above.

The length of this initial phase will depend on the client's response. It will usually last for 2–4 sessions.

Middle stage of therapy

By the end of the first stage the person's emotional distress should be relieved to some extent, and he or she should be familiar with the cognitive model. The middle phase of therapy continues this work within a more explicitly cognitive framework. The aims are:

1. To teach the use of thought monitoring and basic principles of dealing with unhelpful thinking. The Dysfunctional Thoughts Record (DTR) is used as a regular self-help assignment.

2. To continue the process of problem-solving. The focus gradually shifts from the priorities of the first stage—reducing emotional distress and dealing with life crises—to less urgent but equally important issues, such as social isolation, communication problems with partner, difficulty in coping with the unpredictability of cancer. Patient and partner adopt an increasingly active role in problem-solving as therapy progresses.

3. Continuing the process of fighting cancer. Improving quality of life is still a goal, but now cognitive techniques are added to the behavioural techniques. Some patients may wish to explore ways in which they themselves can do things to improve their prognosis.

This stage lasts for 3–6 sessions.

Ending therapy

By the end of the middle stage patient and partner have learned new ways of engaging in life and countering negative thoughts. All the problems may not be totally resolved, but the couple will have the means to continue the process beyond therapy. The final stage looks to the future in the following ways:

1. *Relapse prevention:* coping strategies are discussed which can be used in the future if the cancer recurs or if other stresses in the person's life threaten to cause emotional disturbance. With selected patients, discussion of cancer recurrence and death may be appropriate.

2. *Planning for the future:* as therapy progresses, provided the prognosis is reasonably good, discussion of goals becomes more long-term. Couples are encouraged to set up realistic goals for 3, 6, or 12 months ahead, and to come up with practical plans for achieving them.

3. *Identifying underlying assumptions and core beliefs:* in some people it may be appropriate to look at the beliefs which give rise to their emotional problems, and to help them change some of the rules they habitually apply to themselves and the world. Many people want to change their lifestyles as a result of the encounter with cancer, e.g. placing less emphasis on work achievement, living more healthily, etc. These positive changes can be discussed at this stage if appropriate.

This stage can last for 1–3 sessions. The extent to which these issues are covered in detail will depend on the person's response to the previous phases of APT.

Illustration of APT

The following case demonstrates some of the basic principles of APT outlined in this chapter. To make the illustration of the techniques clearer, a case is chosen which involved mainly individual therapy. Case descriptions elsewhere in the book will show how APT is used with couples. Susan was a 34-year-old woman with breast cancer who was treated with excision biopsy followed by radiotherapy. Two years later a recurrence was discovered in the same breast with metastatic nodes in the other breast. She was reluctant to have a mastectomy or to undergo chemotherapy, and was started on Tamoxifen. As the size of the tumour increased despite hormone treatment she eventually agreed to chemotherapy, receiving three courses of different combination therapies without improvement. She became anxious about the effects of further treatment on her appearance, particularly fearing the loss of her hair. Susan felt increasingly irritable, depressed, and lethargic, and asked to be referred for psychological help. At interview she had a mildly depressed mood, with symptoms of loss of motivation and pleasure, indecisiveness and ruminations about cancer. In particular she was preoccupied with the effects of cancer on her appearance. A diagnosis of mild reactive depression with anxiety was made. Therapy consisted of 12 weekly sessions of APT. She was seen with her husband for the first session, but he was only able to attend on one other occasion despite attempts to engage him.

Beginning therapy

Problems identified in the first session were:

1 Depressed mood.
2 Preoccupation with loss of attractiveness, and mistrust of husband.
3 Marital conflict.

   One of the first goals was relief of her depressed mood. She remarked: 'It's just as if everything I've planned I haven't been able to do … why plan anything?' The therapist encouraged her to express her feelings of anger and hopelessness. While showing empathy for her sadness over the very real losses caused by cancer, the therapist challenged the absolute nature of these statements. These negative thoughts and her loss of motivation became the focus for helping her to concentrate on living an ordinary life. The therapist challenged her belief that there was no point in doing anything by getting her to identify things she was still able to plan. Activities were found which still gave her pleasure and realistic goals were set as homework for the next week, e.g. buying Christmas presents and going out with a friend. She was thus able to gain control over some ordinary areas of her life which had not been affected by cancer. Negative automatic thoughts such as the one described above were elicited early in therapy and used to demonstrate the cognitive model. Activity scheduling continued over the first four sessions, and this helped to increase Susan's mood and motivation.

Middle stage of therapy

In subsequent sessions Susan learned how to identify automatic thoughts herself. She began to monitor automatic thoughts on occasions when she felt depressed or anxious. For instance, while they were in a supermarket one day her husband joked with a shop assistant. She immediately thought: 'He's flirting with her. What a cheek … what does he get up to when I'm not with him?' This made her feel insecure and deserted. Her negative thoughts then continued: 'He's going to leave me eventually! I might as well leave him first'. On examination it seemed she had been sensitized to rejection by an experience of her husband getting cold feet before her wedding, but subsequently her husband had been supportive and shown no signs of wanting to leave. She could not remember any time since their marriage when he had flirted with anyone. She was encouraged to continue this process of reality testing and to substitute more realistic thoughts when she started worrying that he was going to leave. During this part of therapy, she continued the process of trying to live a normal life, and found it useful to make concrete plans on a weekly basis.

Ending therapy

Towards the end of therapy the assumption underlying her negative thoughts was discovered. Susan believed that she could only be of value if she was sexually attractive. She was encouraged to examine whether attractiveness really referred solely to physical appearance or whether it might apply to other characteristics. She was helped by the idea that it was only part of her body which looked different, and in fact in her daily life she looked no different from usual because she had not suffered any major side-effects from chemotherapy. She found that her mood improved as a result of APT, while there was some reduction in her need to base her self-esteem solely on her physical appearance.

Practical considerations

The following chapters consider the methods and format of cognitive behaviour therapy for people with cancer in more detail. Before moving on to the techniques it may be helpful to cover some of the practical matters which need to be taken into account when embarking on a course of therapy. Table 5.1 summarizes the problems that are suitable for therapy together with those conditions for which APT is contraindicated. Beyond this it is difficult to say who is most likely to benefit from treatment. Patients with early disease and relatively good prognosis may well respond best, since these patients can test their negative thoughts about cancer against the touchstone of a realistically good future. This does not mean that patients with advanced disease cannot do well. Studies of group CBT in advanced cancer have shown promising results (Edmonds *et al.* 1999; Edelman *et al.* 1999b) and our own study comparing APT with counselling included a significant proportion of people with metastatic cancer (Moorey *et al.* 1998). Fighting spirit in these cases means optimizing the quality of life, as in the case of Susan, rather than looking forward to cure.

APT is usually given over 6–12 sessions. Many patients do well in the shorter course of treatment, but some require the full 12 sessions. When considering taking therapy beyond six sessions the degree to which the patient's symptoms have been relieved should be taken into account, together with the extent to which patient and partner have learned the principles and techniques of APT. Early symptom improvements in the absence of any evidence that coping strategies have been learned may lead to recurrence of psychological distress. When cancer activates core negative beliefs about the self and the world that are derived from early life experiences, it may not be possible to produce major changes in a few sessions. Therapy then needs to extend for a longer period and much of the work involves understanding how beliefs that the world is a dangerous, abusive place arose, and how cancer confirmed these beliefs, so that less destructive views can be explored and acted on.

Chapter 6

The therapy session

Although the therapist–patient relationship and structure of therapy are often referred to as non-specific aspects of treatment, they are actually essential to the successful use of more specific interventions. This chapter will show how both are necessary for effective cognitive behaviour therapy. Important aspects of the therapeutic relationship covered are:

- warmth, genuineness, and empathy from the therapist;
- the fostering of a partnership to test thoughts and beliefs (collaborative empiricism); and
- the use of guided discovery to question thoughts and beliefs.

Cognitive behaviour therapy puts more emphasis on structuring sessions than other therapies. In this chapter we present:

- how to structure the first session, including establishing rapport, defining problems and goals, explaining the model and setting the first homework;
- how to structure subsequent sessions;
- basic principles of agenda setting;
- the value of frequent summarizing;
- the importance of eliciting feedback.

The therapeutic relationship

The same basic interpersonal skills are needed in APT as in any other form of psychotherapy. The patient needs to feel that he or she is understood. An interested, committed therapist will be more appreciated than an aloof one. If a good therapeutic relationship does not exist techniques such as challenging negative thoughts may appear confrontational and cold. It is therefore vital that the technology does not get in the way of the relationship between patient and therapist.

The role of warmth, genuineness, and empathy in psychotherapy has been intensively investigated. Despite much work the original hypothesis that this is a necessary and sufficient condition of effective treatment has not been sustained (Parloff *et al.* 1978). Most clinicians regard these factors as important but not exclusively significant in producing change. People with cancer need to feel that their therapist has understood something of what they have been going through and is genuinely interested in them as people and their well-being. Burns and Auerbach (1996) reviewed the role of therapeutic empathy in cognitive behaviour therapy, and concluded that the effects of therapeutic empathy on recovery from depression are large 'even in a highly technical form of therapy such as cognitive therapy'. A working alliance in which the patient trusts the therapist and is prepared to discuss and explore painful thoughts and feelings is very important in therapy. Although it is easy to see when a therapist has achieved this kind of rapport, it is more difficult to specify what behaviours are needed to achieve it. Many of the techniques described in Chapter 7 can help the development of rapport. APT, like Beck's cognitive therapy, fosters a therapeutic relationship in which patient and therapist are partners in problem solving. Two essential components of this partnership are 'collaborative empiricism' and 'guided discovery'.

Collaborative empiricism

Beck has coined this term to describe the special relationship which develops in cognitive therapy. Therapy is empirical because it is constantly setting up and testing hypotheses. It is collaborative because the patient is actively involved in this process, helping to define problems and devise solutions both inside and outside the session. There are distinct advantages to this approach. By using the empirical model, the patient's negative *beliefs* are turned into *hypotheses* which can then be tested.

A belief that a patient cannot regain her old sense of control over her life becomes a prediction that she will not be able to overcome feeling helpless:

> I can understand that at the moment it seems you will never be able to get back to your old self after everything you have been through. I know of many people who have been able to make something of their lives in these circumstances, but you may well be different from them. Since neither of us can foretell the future, perhaps we could test out your beliefs by trying an experiment. Would you be willing to try some of the things that other people have found useful in overcoming their feelings of helplessness?

A belief that the cancer might come back at any time and therefore must be guarded against at all costs can be reframed as a prediction that checking for signs of recurrence every day is the best coping strategy:

> At the moment you are checking that the cancer hasn't come back every day. You say that doing this helps to reassure you as well as make sure you pick up a recurrence as soon as possible. Perhaps we could examine whether all the checking you are doing is as helpful as it seems.

Collaborative empiricism allows the therapist to acknowledge that the patient's view of the world makes sense. Giving up if everything seems hopeless, or checking if you fear secondary spread are perfectly sensible behaviours within the patients' belief systems. Rather than taking the belief at face value the therapist helps the patients look for evidence of its accuracy and usefulness. Some people take well to this model. Therapy then becomes a truly collaborative venture, in which the patient can be as creative the therapist in devising methods for coping.

Guided discovery

One of the best methods for helping someone test their thoughts and beliefs is through guided discovery. Asking questions to clarify what the person believes and what evidence there is to support the belief is a much more acceptable and effective way to change attitudes than persuasion. Many negative thoughts about cancer are true whereas others may be distorted or unhelpful. Asking questions enables the patient to sort the realistic from unrealistic thoughts without giving the impression that all negative thoughts are somehow 'wrong'. When working with life-threatening illness it is always better to adopt a stance of inquiry rather than disputation. Guided discovery should lead the person to ask whether there might be an alternative, more constructive view of the situation which could help them fight cancer better. It alternates questions with empathic statements summarizing the person's thoughts and feelings, and should help the patient synthesize all the information about the problem into the most adaptive evaluation. Here is an example of how guided discovery can be used with a patient who is feeling helpless:

Therapist: What makes you think there's no point in trying?

Patient: It just seems never ending, I've seen all those other patients coming back again.

Therapist: Does anything in particular go through your mind when you see that happen?

Patient: Yes, I keep thinking I'll be just the same.

Therapist: That must be a horrible feeling, just the inevitability of it.

Patient: Yes, that's how it feels, inevitable.

Therapist: Did the people you are thinking of have the same type of cancer as you?

Patient: Yes, one of them did.

Therapist: Do you know anyone else who had your type of cancer, but didn't go through many hospital admissions?

Patient: Well, perhaps one or two.

Therapist: Do you think more about the people who did well or about the person who had lots of admissions?

Patient: I think a lot more about the person who just kept going into hospital again and again. I know I shouldn't but I just can't help it.

Therapist: What effect does that have?

Patient: It makes me feel even worse.

Therapist: Even more hopeless, as if it really is inevitable?

Patient: Exactly.

Therapist: So you think more about the person who had a rough time, which makes you feel worse, and you sort of assume that you're going to have the same experience. Is that assumption based on anything you know about your own disease or is it based more on the *feeling* you get when you remember your friend?

Patient: I suppose it's the feeling really. I don't have any reason to believe my illness has to go the same way as hers.

Therapist: What do you make of that?

Patient: Well, it looks like I'm assuming that because it *feels* that way its going to *be* that way. It might not be as inevitable as it seems.

The use of questioning is an important component of all the cognitive techniques to be described later.

The structure of APT

Beck's cognitive therapy has a number of structural elements which have been found to be helpful in brief psychotherapy with emotionally distressed patients (Beck 1995). APT incorporates these structural elements in the treatment programme for cancer patients. In the first session there are some special requirements—the patient (and partner) must be engaged, the problems elicited, the rationale of APT explained and the business of therapy begun.

The first session

Since much cognitive behaviour therapy in liaison settings is brief, the first meeting with the patient is very important in getting therapy started on the right footing. We describe an approach to treatment which combines assessment and the start of treatment at the first meeting. This has certain advantages since it allows the business of learning to cope with problems to be started straight away. The first session may last from an hour to an hour-and-a-half. This method does not suit all clinicians, and some prefer to carry out a full and detailed assessment before instituting any therapy. Both of these approaches are compatible with APT. We describe here how to use the first session as a therapeutic session. Several goals need to be accomplished in this first session.

Establishing rapport

Most people referred for psychological help in oncology have not had any previous contact with psychiatry or psychotherapy. It is therefore vital that they are engaged during the first session or they may not return. The best way to establish rapport is through the use of non-directive counselling techniques and the demonstration of empathy. Listening, reflecting back the patient's statements, and summarizing them succinctly all contribute to the feeling of being understood. As we have said, the fact that APT is a directive, problem-oriented therapy does not lessen the importance of these non-specific factors. They are probably more important than in other cognitive behavioural therapies, because of the relief that patients under stress obtain from expressing their feelings. It is usually helpful to begin by asking the patient to tell something about the way the cancer was discovered, the history of treatment, and to cover relevant aspects of the person's life history. This approach both gathers information and builds rapport by showing an interest in the patient as a person.

Rapport is also established through pursuit of the other goals of the first session. Defining problems helps the patient to feel less overwhelmed and this establishes the therapist's credibility, while explaining the rationale of APT at the outset gives the patient and spouse a framework within which to understand the problems.

Defining problems and goals

As the patient expresses feelings about the experience of cancer, the therapist can help reframe these as a focus for therapy. The starting point must always be the patient and partner's own perceptions of the problems they are facing. These may be symptoms such as depression, anxiety, and irritability or life problems such as financial difficulties, the stage the disease has reached, etc.

In the first interview the couple's thoughts and feelings about the disease should be explored as well as the implications of cancer for the patient's self-image. Information from assessment instruments may be helpful in this process of problem formulation. These assessment questionnaires are reproduced in Appendix V.

1. *The Hospital Anxiety and Depression Scale* (HAD; Zigmond and Snaith 1983) is a 14-item measure of mood which was designed for use with patients with physical illness. Seven items measure anxiety and 7 depression. Its psychometric properties have been investigated in cancer patients (Moorey *et al.* 1991). This scale gives information on the severity of emotional symptoms (cut off scores of 8 for depression and 10 for anxiety indicate clinical cases) and responses to individual questions can point to problems to target.

2. *The Mental Adjustment to Cancer Scale* (MAC; Watson *et al.* 1988) measures styles of adjustment to cancer. The MAC has 5 subscales: fighting spirit, helplessness–hopelessness, anxious preoccupation, fatalism, and positive avoidance. This gives information on the adjustment style the patient is using.

3. *The Concerns Checklist* (Harrison *et al.* 1994) assesses 14 cancer concerns. Patients with 4 or more concerns or who have concerns about sexuality, feeling upset or feeling different are more likely to suffer from anxiety or depression (Harrison *et al.* 1994). Responses to this measure can be used as a starting point for discussion of target problems.

4. *The Cancer Coping Questionnaire* is a 21-item questionnaire designed at the Royal Marsden Hospital to assess the cognitive, behavioural, and interpersonal coping strategies taught in APT. Its reliability and validity have been investigated recently (Moorey *et al.*, unpublished manuscript). Patients' responses to individual questions can give information about coping strengths and deficits.

Typical problems which might be identified are:

- General problems unrelated to cancer type, e.g. feelings of helplessness, the unpredictability of outcome, fears of death and recurrence, treatment.
- Specific problems related to cancer type, e.g. feeling dirty (cancer of the cervix or the bowel), feeling unfeminine (about the breast), worries about sexuality (more common in breast, gynaecological and testicular cancers) etc.

- Emotional disturbance, e.g. depression, anxiety, guilt, anger.
- Interpersonal problems, e.g. arguments with spouse, social isolation, feeling different.
- Physical problems, e.g. lethargy, nausea, pain, inability to do things.
- Socio-economic problems, e.g. job, finances.

Problems cannot all be exhaustively explored, but by the end of the session a list of the most important problems can be drawn up. This exercise in problem definition is the first step in showing patients that they can regain control over some aspects of their lives. Once the list is drawn up the therapist can collaborate with patient and spouse in choosing the problems that are most important. When doing this, account should be taken of the issues which the couple see as a priority. The therapist should also look for problems which can be tackled quickly and effectively. For example, a woman may say her biggest problem is knowing what decisions to make about her child's future. If the patient is depressed this may be too big to deal with early in therapy. It may be better to accept the importance of this but leave it till later, focusing initially on other symptoms such as depressed mood, lack of interest, or hopelessness. When the woman's mood has improved she will feel more able to think about making important decisions.

A 40-year-old woman with carcinoma of the ovary was referred because, although she had an encapsulated tumour which was caught very early, she had great difficulty accepting that her prognosis was good. During the interview she described feeling very hopeless, frequently tearful and tense. She was sure that the cancer was still there, and constantly thought of how it might have spread elsewhere in her body. This was not helped by the fact that she had recently had a liver scan for what was initially thought to be a metastasis but proved to be a benign cyst.

In addition to the cancer, she described other stresses in her life. Her boyfriend was unable to give her a firm commitment in the relationship, her 15-year-old daughter was acting rebelliously, and she was under extreme pressure in her job as a lecturer. She appeared very anxious during the interview and was fidgety and spoke rapidly. The therapist took a background history but focused on her current problems. A problem list was drawn up:

Problem	Goal
1. Anxiety and stress	Learn strategies for dealing with anxiety and stress.
2. Attitude to cancer—hopelessness and anxious pre-occupation	Become more hopeful and get through a week without being preoccupied with cancer.
3. Relationship with boyfriend	*Short term:* Enjoy time with boyfriend without pressuring him. *Longer term:* Make decisions about our relationship.
4. Relationship with a daughter	Be able to spend 2 hours together each week where we have quality time and don't argue.
5. Stresses at work	Manage my workload so that I feel on top of the demands made on me.

The therapist was sensitive to the patient's feeling of being under great pressure and helped her to conceptualize her anxiety symptoms as a response to the stresses she was under from cancer and her life. The first intervention was to teach her anxiety management techniques involving relaxation, and identification of anxiety-provoking thoughts. This focus allowed the therapist to teach the patient coping strategies which could be applied to the various problem areas. Later on in therapy these areas were addressed in their own right.

It is often possible to move from the problem list to goals in the first session. Questions such as, 'How would you know that this problem was solved/reduced?' 'What would need to happen for this problem to be less worrying?' 'Can you think of something that you will be able to do when this problem is alleviated?' elicit realistic, attainable and wherever possible behaviourally defined goals.

Explaining the cognitive model and rationale of therapy

In a short-term therapy much of the emphasis is placed on developing skills which the patient can continue to use when therapy has ended. To use these self-help skills properly the patient must understand their rationale. The basic features of APT are explained in the first session. Automatic thoughts are elicited and the therapist shows the patient how they contribute to his or her emotional distress. Patients will not understand the concepts fully in the first session, but usually they are able to grasp the idea that their thoughts may in some way be contributing to their distress. It is essential that the therapist introduces the key concepts of cognitive therapy: *the way we view situations determines our reactions to them.* Three main points are explained:

1　APT is active, directive and aimed at helping the patient to develop a constructive and positive approach to coping with cancer.

2　APT is based on cognitive therapy. Examples from the patient's own experience are used to show the relationship between thoughts and feelings.

3　The practicalities, i.e. 6–12 sessions, joint meetings, use of self-help assignments, are explained.

The educational process goes on throughout therapy. The patient needs to understand the purpose of each new intervention, whether behavioural or cognitive, and to see how it might be applied in other situations. We will consider how the rationale for various techniques can be explained to the patient when we cover those interventions in succeeding chapters.

The importance of providing some sort of road-map for therapy cannot be underestimated. Fennell and Teasdale (1987) using Beck's cognitive therapy with depressed patients have found that acceptance of the cognitive model predicts response to therapy. They were able to divide patients who received cognitive therapy into rapid and slow responders. Those who responded rapidly were more likely to react positively to the explanation of the cognitive model of depression in the first session, and were also more likely to have a positive response to the first homework assignment. The rationale provides a framework in which the patient and spouse can understand their reactions to cancer, and also offers hope. Patients benefit from reading the booklet *Coping with cancer* (Appendix I). This will usually form part of the first homework assignment and is used to reinforce the educational component of the first session.

The cognitive model at this stage generally just covers the interaction between the patient's thoughts, feelings, mood, and behaviour and demonstrates how the current problems relate to these systems. Drawing a diagram of this interaction may be very helpful, both for therapist and patient. In some cases a deeper conceptualization is possible even from the first session. The individual's core beliefs might come out as very obvious themes from the problem list and history.

Setting homework

In addition to asking the patient to read *Coping with cancer*, the therapist will usually set a homework task designed to attack one of the patient's presenting problems. This will usually be a behavioural task, but may sometimes be a cognitive assignment such as monitoring negative thoughts. Anxious patients can be taught relaxation and then asked to practise this over the following week. Depressed patients often benefit from some structured tasks such as scheduling of pleasant activities, or activities which induce a sense of personal control. In the examples cited above the woman with an anxious preoccupation about her ovarian cancer was given two homework tasks. She was asked to record her experience of stress over the next week in whatever circumstances this occurred. The therapist drew up a chart for her which included sections on degree of stress, the situation in which it occurred an automatic thoughts associated with it (Table 6.1). The second task was to listen to a relaxation tape and if possible to carry out some relaxation exercises each day. She also read *Coping with cancer.*

Not all patients will be able to carry out such a demanding programme. This woman was intelligent and well-educated and very quickly grasped the requirements of therapy. With other patients, and particularly those with more disabling symptoms, the expectations may be more modest. Carrying out a simple task such as visiting a relative maybe all that some patients can be expected to do after the first session.

Table 6.1 Monitoring stressful situations: first homework assignment

Situation	Stress rating (0–10)	Automatic thoughts	Coping response
Boyfriend not arriving on time	7	He wants me to think he is finishing with me. He shouldn't put me under all this stress	Busied myself; watched television
Daughter ate the crisps I was keeping for a party	9	My God, I can't keep anything in the house. She ought to help me more. She's not thinking of me	Drank two glasses of sherry. Yelled at her to get it out of my system

The structure of subsequent sessions

After the first or second session the format settles down to a regular pattern. Feedback from the previous session, the events of the last week, and the success or failure of homework assignments all need to be covered, as well as the main problem the patient wishes to discuss. The usual plan for a therapy session can be summarized as follows:

1 Set agenda. Only one or two topics.
2 Review the patient's week and get feedback from previous session.
3 Review homework. Pick out the main details, e.g. lessons learned or difficulties experienced.
4 Start on main topic of session:
   ◆ define problem clearly;
   ◆ identify associated negative thinking;
   ◆ answer it;
   ◆ work out how to handle the problem differently in the future.
5 Set homework. Make it relevant to the individual and to the content of the session.
6 Ask for feedback.

Although the structure of sessions remains constant, the content will vary depending on the phase of therapy and the nature of the patient and partner's problems.

Agenda-setting

Because APT is a short-term therapy, time is at a premium. The structure of the session allows time to be used effectively by agreeing an agenda with the patient and summarizing particular issues and interventions during the session. The structure of therapy allows flexibility and is not applied rigidly, but is more of a framework. At times it may be necessary to step outside this framework, for instance if the patient has recently been told of a recurrence of the disease and needs to express his or her feelings immediately it may be inappropriate to set a formal agenda. However, by the end of the session, when the patient has ventilated his or her feelings, it is usually possible to reassert the structure by summarizing the content of the session and looking for coping strategies which the patient might try out.

At the beginning of each session the patient and therapist decide on the main topics for discussion. Part of the agenda will contain feedback on the last session, a report on homework, and a brief review of the previous week. The rest of the session is then devoted to the main agenda items. It is usually best to keep to one or two items only. It is also helpful, after starting work on a problem, to continue with that problem at the next session so that significant inroads have been made into it, rather than changing from one problem to another. Once an agenda has been set, it is best to keep to it unless a very important new item, such as suicidal ideas, arises which needs to replace it.

The advantages of agenda-setting are:

1 It allows for a judicious use of the short time available in APT.
2 It helps to model the process of problem definition and problem-solving.

3   The structure provided helps to keep patients on track. This is particularly important for patients whose attention and concentration are impaired by depression or anxiety.

4   If used well, the patient contributes to agenda-setting as part of the collaborative relationship.

Summaries

The therapist makes summaries several times during the course of a session of cognitive behaviour therapy, usually after an important intervention or at the end of an agenda item. This helps to clarify for the therapist and patient what the cognitive conceptualization of the problem is and what methods have been developed to deal with it. A final summary is also useful at the end of the session. Summaries help to keep patient and therapist on track, and aid retention of insights and therapeutic strategies. As therapy progresses the patient becomes increasingly responsible for providing these summaries; this is another way of empowering the patient and finding out how much learning has occurred during the session. A typical capsule summary might be:

> From what we have been discussing today it seems that attractiveness is an important issue for you. We began by looking at situations which make you feel bad and found that they often involve meeting other women. When we examined the thoughts you had in these situations, they all had the theme of comparison. You said: 'She's prettier than me' or 'I hate her *she* hasn't had a mastectomy'. The next step is to see if these thoughts and comparisons are realistic and helpful. Before we do that, could you tell me if I've summarized the problem correctly?

Feedback

Therapeutic alliance can only be built up if the professional has a clear idea about the client's perception of the problem, the therapy, and the therapist. Surprisingly, traditional psychotherapy has not paid much attention to gathering information systematically about the patient's reactions to particular interventions in therapy. APT makes use of regular feedback, both at the end of each session and at strategic points during the session. Asking for feedback also helps to prevent difficulties in the therapeutic relationship. On the whole, transference is not a focus in this type of therapy, so wherever possible collaborative therapeutic relationship is encouraged so that a problem-solving approach prevails. Distorted thoughts about the therapist or therapy can get in the way of this.

> A woman who had been treated for malignant melanoma 12 months previously had developed an anxious preoccupation with the disease. Although there were no signs of recurrence she could think of nothing else. During the first session she initially showed great relief at being able to talk about her anxieties to a sympathetic listener. The therapist gradually led her to the point where he asked about her fears of death, of which she talked reluctantly. Later on in the session she changed her attitude dramatically and asserted that she was all right now and would get better. When the therapist tried to talk about some strategies for managing her anxiety she became very angry. It emerged, after the therapist

asked her for feedback on his effect on her, that she had perceived the questions as being too negative. She only wanted to hear good things about cancer and believed the therapist was acting wrongly in apparently forcing her to think about her fears. This problem might have been prevented if the therapist had been more sensitive to her emotional change during the session and asked for feedback earlier.

Feedback frequently reveals that the client's idea of what was useful in the session is very different from the therapist's, which is a salutary finding. Feedback also reveals stumbling blocks to between-session assignments. Automatic thoughts like; 'I'll never do it', 'What's the point?' or 'It won't work' are common responses to homework assignments, but the patient often only expresses these thoughts if asked specifically. Once they are identified these thoughts can be challenged within the collaborative relationship.

Summary

In cognitive behaviour therapy, like all psychotherapies, the personal skills of the therapist form the basis upon which a therapeutic relationship is established. Skills in listening, reflecting, and showing empathy are used in everyday life; some people find it easier to use them than others. In addition to these basic skills cognitive behaviour therapy fosters a particular type of relationship which involves collaboration in solving problems, where the therapist helps the patient to test beliefs through a process of guided discovery. This collaborative empiricism allows the patient and partner to develop their skills as 'personal scientists'. The collaborative relationship is embedded in a structured therapy session which uses agenda-setting, summaries, and regular feedback to maximize the alliance between patient and therapist in learning new skills for coping with cancer. Whatever the techniques employed, whether they are cognitive, behavioural, or emotive, the structured, collaborative therapy session is a hallmark of cognitive behaviour therapy.

Chapter 7

Experiencing and expressing emotions in adjuvant psychological therapy

As we have seen in the first part of this book, learning that you have a potentially fatal illness can shatter your assumptions about your world and yourself. Reconstructing your world-view requires both cognitive and emotional processing, yet at times the sheer enormity of the threat and the raw emotions experienced can be overwhelming. Horowitz (1986) postulates two oscillating phases in the adjustment process: one of 'overmodulated' emotions where avoidance and denial are manifest, and another of 'undermodulated' emotions where overwhelming feelings are experienced. The person facing a trauma moves between these emotional states as the system tries to regulate affect so that the new information can be incorporated into old schemas, or new schemas can be formed. The behavioural and cognitive techniques in Chapters 8, 9, and 10 are mainly aimed at helping people to regulate negative emotions. This chapter discusses how emotions can be shut down when the impact of cancer becomes too threatening. The mechanisms of avoidance of emotional experiencing are described, and also the way in which people often try to supress strong feelings. The importance of acknowledging and expressing emotions in the adjustment process is considered.

We present the following clinical skills:

 • when to facilitate emotions and when to help the person to regulate them;
 • how to facilitate emotional experiencing and emotional expression;
 • working with denial;
 • methods for helping people to ventilate and channel anger.

Avoidance of negative emotions

From a cognitive perspective three different processes may operate to prevent us experiencing strong emotions in the face of objectively distressing events. These are cognitive distortion, cognitive avoidance, and affective avoidance.

We have already introduced the concept of cognitive distortion in its negative form (page 18) and we have also talked of our tendency to operate a slight positive bias (page 18). For instance, Weinstein (1980; Weinstein and Lachendro 1982) demonstrated that people overestimate the likelihood of experiencing positive outcomes in life and underestimate the likelihood of experiencing negative events.

This positive bias may shift imperceptibly from an optimistic view (which we call fighting spirit) to an objectively unrealistic optimism (which we call denial). Many people with cancer persist in thinking they will be cured against all the odds. They may deny that their illness is life-threatening. In extreme forms they may even deny that they have cancer at all. As was described in Chapter 2, this denial can be considered as a negative schema which makes sense of the cancer and the threat to survival. Cognitive distortion minimizes the impact of the disease. In denial, cognitive distortion operates in an unrealistically positive way, whereas in the other adjustment styles the distortions are usually negative. The consequence of attending exclusively to the good news you hear and excluding the bad news is that you reduce the perceived threat and so avoid painful emotions.

We encountered an example of this positive distortion when testing a coping measure in our research some years ago. A 60-year-old woman with cancer of the cervix had undergone a radical vulvectomy. She had a colostomy and urostomy, but despite all this appeared very cheerful. She scored low on the coping questionnaire because she did not feel in the least stressed and did not feel there were any problems with which she needed to cope. She did not consider that her operations had caused any difficulties in her life at all, reporting spontaneously how she had been very amused when her grandson had said 'You're very lucky, granny, you can go to the toilet and go shopping all at the same time'. This woman was selectively filtering out all the negative aspects of her disease. She did not see it as a challenge or a threat, but a minor irritant.

A second way to avoid painful feelings is to focus attention elsewhere. Cognitive avoidance occurs when the person voluntarily or automatically avoids thoughts and images which might cause distress. This is a process we all use at times—focusing on other topics, distracting ourselves, saying: 'It's best not to think about it'—and it can be an adaptive coping strategy. At other times it is only partly effective and the negative emotions break through, but the patient does not have immediate access to the cognitions that produce the feelings. An example of this might be a man with cancer of the larynx who cries inexplicably while watching television. He may have no idea why he feels so upset. Further probing of the situation might reveal that he was watching a programme in which a man argued with his wife and shouted at her. This reminded him of how difficult he found communicating strong emotions following laryngectomy. Cognitions like: 'I can't have a good row anymore', or 'I can't get across how I feel', may have occurred at the time, but he rapidly avoided them.

The final form of avoidance, affective avoidance is a dissociative mechanism in which the person blocks off painful emotions. The patient is able to talk about distressing events without any emotional reaction. This may sometimes protect the person from painful feelings, but often this dissociation may be associated with somatic symptoms such as headaches, dizziness, etc. The woman who had a vulvectomy was practising affective avoidance when she discussed realistically the effects of her operation but did not have any associated feelings.

Positively biasing perception and interpretation, distracting oneself from painful thoughts and dissociating from painful emotions can all be healthy ways of shutting down when feelings become too overwhelming. They are part of the overmodulation of affect necessary in the emotional processing of traumatic events. They should not lead to therapeutic intervention unless they cause significant problems for the patient or the family. We will consider how to deal with denial later in the chapter.

Suppression and expression of negative emotions

Many people experience appropriate negative emotions but do not express them openly. There are several factors which make acknowledging and expressing emotions difficult for someone with cancer. The patient's position is one of relative helplessness, making it difficult to show anger or fight in the sick role. Fears of abandonment by professionals, relatives, or friends if they are perceived as difficult or 'bolshy' can prevent people from showing how scared or angry they really feel. Altruistic motives can also contribute to emotional suppression in this situation: selflessness based on the concern that caregivers have so much to cope with they should not be burdened with negative emotions. There has long been an impression that people with cancer seem to supress emotions and are more likely to subjugate their own needs to those of other people. There is some support for this clinical impression. Fernandez-Ballesteros *et al.* (1998) compared 311 women with breast cancer with 103 healthy women. Women with breast cancer had higher scores on 'anti-emotionality' as measured by the Rationality/Emotional Defensiveness Scale and were ready to sacrifice their needs to achieve and maintain harmonious relationships (measured by the Need for Harmony Scale). Servaes *et al.* (1999) compared 48 women with breast cancer with 49 healthy women with respect to alexithymia (an inability to express emotion), emotional expression, assertiveness, repression, and distress. No difference was found between the two groups in alexithymia, expressing emotions or willingness to talk with others about emotions generally. However, the patient group were more ambivalent about emotional expression and showed more restraint. They report that 'the image of the breast cancer patient that emerged in the study was that of a person who has conflicting feelings with regard to expressing emotions, is reserved and anxious, is self-effacing, and represses aggression and impulsiveness.' They conclude that emotional inhibition is a reaction to the disease rather than a personality trait. Conflicting evidence does exist, suggesting that this inhibition may be more of a state than a trait feature and that suppression of emotions may be of aetiological significance in cancer (Greer and Morris 1975), and may also be related to disease outcome (Temoshok *et al.* 1985). Whatever the underlying cause of emotional suppression, it does seem to be associated with poorer adjustment to cancer. Stanton *et al.* (2000a) studied 92 women with breast cancer immediately after medical treatment and then 3 months later. Those who coped through expressing emotions had less distress and better physical health and vigour over the next 3 months. One possibility is that expressive coping acts as a vehicle for energizing active coping and fighting spirit.

The value of emotional expression

It is too simplistic to assert that expressing emotions is therapeutic in its own right. Although catharsis is often described as one of the basic ingredients in psychotherapy (Frank 1971) research in this area is not conclusive. Ventilation of feelings or catharsis only seems to be effective if it is accompanied by cognitive processing (Lewis and

Bucher 1992). One line of research, carried out by Pennebaker and colleagues (Smyth and Pennebaker 1999) provides compelling evidence that talking or writing about stressful experiences has benefits for health. Lumley *et al.* (1997) examined the effects of emotional disclosure on the clinical state of people with rheumatoid arthritis. At three months people who had disclosed about past trauma had less affective distur-bance and better physical functioning than those who disclosed about neutral topics. In the field of psychotherapy, where the value of ventilation of feelings has always been recognized, even humanistic therapists are recognizing that emoting is only use-ful when it is connected with cognitive and behavioural change. Greenberg and Safran (1987) consider that the creation of new meaning when feelings are authenti-cally experienced, owned and expressed is a vital component of therapeutic change. They also see emotions as acting to facilitate problem solving by directing us towards constructive action. This link between emotional engagement and adaptive coping behaviour is present in the concept of emotional approach coping (Stanton *et al.* 2000b). Emotional approach coping implies an active confrontation of thoughts and feelings about cancer. This correlates positively with hope (Stanton *et al.* 2000a) a construct described by Stanton as reflecting 'a sense of goal-directed determination, and ability to generate planes to achieve goals.' No research has yet been carried out on emotional approach coping in relation to 'fighting spirit', but we would predict there would be a similar positive association. Thus acknowledging and expressing feelings is integrally connected with construing the situation in a new way, and devel-oping appropriate plans for coping with the stress. Cognitive change takes place most effectively in the presence of affective arousal.

It is our clinical impression that giving patients the opportunity to tell their story is often one of the most important aspects of therapy. People who are going through the process of adjustment to their diagnosis or who are coming to terms with a new development such as a recurrence benefit from having time just to express their feel-ings. Social factors may have operated to prevent them from talking through their thoughts and feelings about cancer. Patients who are socially isolated have no one to talk to, patients who are in poor marriages do not feel supported enough to express themselves, and as we have suggested, many patients in good relationships do not want to burden their family. Studies have shown that a high proportion of people with cancer (86% in a study by Mitchell and Glickman in 1977) wish that they could discuss their situation more fully with someone.

Processing or problem solving?

Although many patients benefit from ventilation of feelings, there are others who have spent a considerable amount of time doing just that, but with little or no benefit. Indeed, the cognitive model would predict that talking about negative feelings will make one feel worse unless there is some reconstrual of the situation. Cancer patients who are depressed or anxious are often stuck in repetitive negative thoughts which they cannot re-evaluate. The challenge in working with this group of patients is to find the right balance between 'doing to' and 'being with' the person, between focusing on acceptance or change, and between facilitating emotional processing and encouraging active problem solving. As a general rule when affect is overmodulated, emotional engagement and expression is required but when affect is undermodulated cognitive and behavioural techniques are needed. Wiser and Arnow (2001) have recently proposed some guidelines for when emotional expression should be facilitated in psychotherapy and when it should not. Moorey (1996) suggested some factors to consider when deciding whether or not to encourage ventilation in people facing adverse life circumstances. The primary consideration is whether the person is going through a process of adjustment or is caught in a persistent negative mood state. If there is evidence for a continuing or arrested adjustment reaction, then emotive techniques may be appropriate. If however, the person is markedly anxious or depressed, or if they might have difficulty in tolerating high levels of emotional arousal, more problem oriented techniques are indicated.

Indications for facilitating emotional expression

- Recent onset of emotional distress in setting of specific change in cancer status (e.g. diagnosis, recurrence, check-up)
- Markedly fluctuating emotional reactions
- Presence of primary emotions—sadness not depression, fear not anxiety
- Absence of cognitive disorders—thought content negative but appropriate
- Significant beliefs about the negative impact of expressing emotions

Indications for problem focused interventions

- Prolonged negative mood state—anxiety, depression, anger
- Affect overwhelming for patient
- Significant behavioural deficits (e.g. prolonged periods in bed because of depressed mood) or behavioural avoidance (e.g. phobia of chemotherapy)
- Presence of maladaptive emotions and cognitive distortions—guilt, self blame, persuasive hopelessness.

Facilitating emotional expression

In practice the distinction between ventilation and problem solving is not so clear cut. It is always necessary to help the person to engage with their feelings and express them before using cognitive or behavioural interventions. Without this it is impossible to understand the personal meaning of the situation for the patient. The therapist acknowledges the fact that any negative feeling is real for the patient, no matter how unrealistic it may be. This validation is important in establishing and maintaining the therapeutic alliance. The feeling must be acknowledged before moving on to the cognitive content of the problem. There is some empirical evidence that a good therapeutic alliance combined with emotional involvement (experiencing) from the patient is associated with better outcome in CBT for depression (Castonguay *et al.* 1996). There is also evidence that some therapist interventions are more likely to help patients maintain a state of high emotional experiencing in CBT (Wiser and Goldfried 1998).

A number of things can be done to encourage experiencing of appropriate affect (see Greenberg and Safran (1987) for more detailed discussion):

+ Educate the patient about emotional reactions to cancer (normalization).
+ Be less active, simply being silent for a while may allow feelings to emerge.
+ Use open ended, rather than closed questions.
+ Use reflective comments such as 'I can understand how you feel'.
+ Attend, and help patient attend, to emotionally relevant experience—'What is that like for you now?' 'How do you feel?'
+ Pay attention to the patient's manner of expression, facial and postural expressions, sighs etc.
+ Keep the focus to experiencing in the here and now.
+ Use the 'poignancy criterion'—if the material feels poignant for the therapist it is probably relevant to appropriate emotional expression.
+ When patient moves to third person language bring them back to first person— 'You feel …'
+ Challenge negative thoughts and beliefs about emotional expression (Moorey 1996).

Getting the patient to accept negative emotions can often break into the circle of distress he or she is experiencing. Teasdale (1983) describes how people can get 'depressed about depression' by focusing on symptoms such as tiredness, lack of concentration, or lack of pleasurable activities. Clinical experience suggests that this applies to the person with cancer, and is not just restricted to depression. Patients frequently report that they feel guilty over their increased irritation and angry outbursts. If they can accept their anger this may defuse the situation considerably. Accepting emotions can also allow patients to step back and observe themselves more objectively. Various methods can be used by the patient:

+ Counting to 10 or taking a deep breath before acting on the feeling, or trying to avoid it.
+ Saying: 'this is a normal feeling, there is nothing wrong with feeling angry/frightened/sad'.
+ Imagining that the emotion is like a wave. The patient is a surfer who rides the wave until it is gone.

The following example, taken from a first session of APT, demonstrates how the therapist can identify possible areas of emotional significance from the cues the patient presents. The patient was a 55-year-old woman who had carcinoma of the cervix. As part of the assessment the therapist had asked about her family.

Patient: I've got no family of my own.

Therapist: Why is that, have your parents died?

Patient: Yes. My brother's; I don't see anything of him and that's that.

(Therapist here sensed that she was resentful of her brother not visiting. This statement, together with the first 'I've got no family of my own', suggested that the patient felt alone and deserted.)

Therapist: How long ago did your parents die?

Patient: My dad died five years ago, and my mum's been gone 13 years now.

Therapist: (Sensing from the patient's non-verbal reaction of looking tense and sad that this was still a significant loss). Were you very close to them?

Patient: Yeah (looking tearful).

Therapist: And you still miss them (emphatically stating the patient's feeling of loss).

Patient: (Nods, sobbing.)

Therapist: Just talking about it makes you feel upset.

Patient: That is one problem I never sorted out. That is the problem, you've hit it on the head.

Therapist: Who do you miss most?

Patient: My mother (sobbing).

Therapist: Your mother (repeating patient's own words).

Patient: I nursed her till she died … I did everything for her and it was her that I miss terribly. I never got over her death.

Having elicited this strong emotional reaction, the therapist was able to explore the meaning of this loss and to make some hypotheses about why it was still so vivid. Two significant factors seemed to emerge. Firstly, the mother had been very close, and despite a long illness with cirrhosis of the liver provided great emotional support to the patient. In the second session the therapist asked how her mother might have helped her to cope. The patient replied: 'She would have worried about it for me. She would have told me it was going to be all right'. Her mother had shouldered all her burdens and reassured her.

The therapist needed to construct a plan of action which both helped the woman to learn some coping strategies for herself, and also used her social support network, since it was unlikely that she was going to give up her dependence needs that easily. The second factor was the resonance that the patient's illness had set up with memories of her mother's death. Expressing her feelings about this gave her a sense of relief, particularly admitting her own fears of a long, lingering death.

Sometimes catharsis occurs later in therapy around a key issue. Jenny, whose case is described in Chapter 8, was helped by being allowed to express some of her fears about her child's future. Halfway through treatment she visited a colleague in hospital. This woman also had cancer and was dying. Jenny handled the situation extremely well at the time but had a delayed reaction to it later and got quite upset.

When we explored this during the therapy session she spoke of her feelings of identification with her friend and her fears of death. The therapist encouraged her to express her negative feelings openly and she cried for the first time in treatment. Her main fears undoubtedly concerned her son and his future. She described feeling guilty 'for doing such a terrible thing to him'. She also worried about his future development if she died. And the therapist used empathy and reflection both to let her talk about this and to experience the emotions associated with it. This in itself was helpful; she had probably been thinking about it but was hesitant to face up to it.

Later in the session the therapist helped her to clarify her realistic sadness at the thought of leaving her son, and to distinguish this from the distorted thinking associated with her guilt. She quickly saw that she could not hold herself responsible for the cancer or the effect of her death on her child, but she could do all in her power to make sure that his future was provided for. The session ended with a review of the objective factors of her disease—that she had early breast cancer which had been successfully treated—to help her continue with her fight against the disease.

Working with denial

Denial is not automatically challenged in APT since it may be an adaptive way of coping. If there are objective signs that the distorted positive thinking is harming the patient it should be tackled using the techniques for encouraging emotional expression described above and the techniques of reality testing described in Chapter 9. Some of the situations in which it might be necessary to challenge denial are:

- When denial of the existence or seriousness of cancer prevents the patient from engaging in treatment.
- When the patient's or spouse's denial causes such a mismatch in their perception of the disease that communication problems and emotional distress occur.
- When denial is not an effective coping strategy and breakthrough anxiety or depression occurs.
- When denial prevents active problem-solving, e.g. a dying man does not make necessary plans for the future of his family.

Encouraging and channelling expression of anger

As with denial, anger can be addressed through emotion-based and cognitive behavioural techniques. Some of the techniques for challenging angry thoughts are described in Chapter 10. Here we present some ways to encourage expression of appropriate anger and to channel it constructively.

Ventilation

When a patient perceives the situation as unjust, the emotional reaction will tend to be one of anger. Most people will find some way of expressing this openly, or will at least accept the emotion. The person who supresses anger feels that it is unsafe, or even morally wrong, to get angry. Cognitive avoidance may also come into play to prevent the person attending to the thoughts associated with this negative affect, so there may be denial of the anger. The cognitive processes associated with the perceived insult will, however, continue to operate. A self-destructive smouldering resentment may then be set up.

In many situations merely expressing the anger may be therapeutic in its own right. Ventilation may be easier than trying to challenge the irrational basis of the anger, since this implicitly reinforces the injunction against angry feelings. Simply telling someone you're angry with him can prevent the resentment from escalating. For those who bottle up feelings it may be helpful to set aside times when they can be 'emotional'. Once ventilation has produced some emotional relief, it is possible to examine the cognition associated with the emotion and find alternative ways of dealing with it in the future.

Positive action

It is not always possible to express anger openly. If anger is felt towards God or the boss it is possible to express this face-to-face. Activities that allow the person to let off steam can be planned, e.g. Going jogging, punching a pillow, etc. An alternative to letting off steam is to adopt a problem-solving approach. The energy from the anger can be channelled or 'sublimated' into action which overcomes the perceived problem. For instance, if the patient says: 'The doctor didn't give me enough chance to ask questions', there are a number of actions the patient can take to achieve the goal of finding out certain things he or she wants to know. The doctor can be confronted directly, or alternatively other sources of information can be consulted. It may be necessary to teach the patient assertiveness skills in order to achieve the goal of the positive action. Unassertive people may quickly change from anger to helplessness in the way they construe a situation. Getting them to do something to overcome the obstacle is a means of increasing self-efficacy. More behavioural and cognitive techniques for dealing with anger are found in Chapter 10.

Summary

Despite the emphasis on cognitions and behaviour, APT places great importance on emotions. Emotions, cognitions, and behaviour are integrally connected in the adjustment process. Negative emotions need to be experienced and expressed in order to process the trauma of a life-threatening illness cognitively and emotionally. We have presented some guidelines for when emotional processing should be encouraged and when it is more appropriate to pursue a problem focus. Techniques for facilitating emotional expression and for working with denial and anger have been described. In the next two chapters we address the behavioural and cognitive components of this cognitive-behavioural-affective system.

Chapter 8

Behavioural techniques

The primary aim of the behavioural interventions in APT is to enable the patient to make maximum use of the activities available within the constraints of the disease. This helps to foster a fighting spirit and a sense of personal control. Behavioural techniques can also be used to cope with stress (relaxation training), and as a means of changing attitudes (behavioural experiments). Since this is a *cognitive* behavioural therapy, behaviour change is usually designed to test specific thoughts or beliefs. Ideally these interventions should come from the conceptualization of the person's problems. For instance, the meaning of cancer for one woman was that she was now alone and isolated. The therapist helped her to test this belief by asking her to contact friends and assess their reactions to her invitation to meet. She found that although some said they were busy, or sounded uncomfortable in talking to her because of her illness, most were very pleased to hear from her and eager to help in any way they could. In other cases, behavioural techniques may be directed at alleviating anxiety or depression. The rationale for any intervention should always be explained to the patient, and incorporated within the shared conceptualization. Behavioural tasks are collaboratively developed as homework assignments. They may be suggested as methods to distract the patient from negative thoughts, test unhelpful beliefs or build feelings of self-efficacy. The patient must understand the rationale for any assignment in order to increase the chances of the assignment being carried out.

In this chapter we present the following behavioural techniques:

- relaxation training
- activity scheduling
- graded task assignment
- planning for the future
- behavioural experiments.

Illustrations are given of how to work behaviourally with threats to survival in anxiously preoccupied and hopeless patients, and how to deal with anxiety and depression that arises from threats to self-image and self-esteem.

Relaxation training

Anxiety is one of the commonest symptoms among people with cancer. In the cognitive model this emotion results from the recognition of a significant threat to survival or to the view of the self and the world, combined with a reduction in the confidence that there are resources available to cope with the threat. Since the disease is genuinely life-threatening and no-one can be certain that their own resources or the treatment they receive will guarantee cure, anxiety is a realistic and natural reaction. What might be termed 'normal' anxiety merges imperceptibly into pathological anxiety. The extent to which anxiety symptoms are a focus in therapy is determined by their severity in relation to the objective threats of cancer, their duration and interference with everyday life, and whether or not the patient sees them as a problem.

Relaxation does not have to be confined to regular sessions at home. It can be used as a coping device in stressful situations. Patients can be taught to relax whenever they feel tense or anxious. Breathing exercises may be more helpful than muscle relaxation since they can be done when the patient is sitting or walking. The therapist needs to analyse the anxiety-provoking situation and find cues that can act as reminders of when to relax. The patient then practises relaxing on cue in the session. These exercises can then be combined with distraction, self-instruction, and cognitive restructuring to produce an anxiety management package tailored for each patient. Situations in which this might be used include waiting for and undergoing radiotherapy or chemotherapy, and going into new social situations.

Relaxation training is a simple, effective and rapid method for giving people control of their anxiety symptoms. Two forms of relaxation are taught: progressive muscle relaxation and breathing exercises. Research suggests that these are equally effective, but individual patients may prefer one to the other. People who have pulmonary problems or suffer from shortness of breath may not find breathing the best focus for relaxation training. Imagery techniques can prove a useful method for these patients.

The exercises described below are instructions to patients from the handbook developed by the Beth Israel Hospital (Borysenko *et al.* 1986). They can be used as a guide to teaching patients the two types of relaxation.

Progressive muscle relaxation

Each of the following tension/relaxation exercises is done in conjunction with the breathing. Tense each body part to its maximum as you breathe in. Hold it as long as it is comfortable. Let go of tension gradually as you exhale.

- Make fists with your toes. Relax.
- Pull the feet back, bringing the toes towards the knees. Relax.
- Tense the muscles of the thighs as if you were trying to lift your legs against a weight. Relax.
- Pinch the buttocks in and up, making them hard. It is as if you were seated upon a rock. Relax.
- Take a big chest breath and pull the abdomen in, hardening it. Relax.
- Take a big chest breath and tense the whole upper-body. Relax
- Make fists with your hands. Relax.
- Pull your hands back at the wrists, as if to bend the hand up towards the elbow. Relax.

+ Raise your shoulders up to your ears. Relax.
+ Raise your eyebrows and furrow your forehead. Relax.
+ Squeeze your eyes shut. Relax.
+ Smile, pulling back the corners of the mouth and baring your teeth. Relax.

Breathing exercises

1. *Awareness of breathing*: as you continue your activities, become aware of your breathing. Inhale deeply, exhale completely and focus attention on belly-breathing. This exercise can be a short as one breath or as long as several minutes.

2. *10–1 countdown*: close your eyes. Take a deep breath and exhale completely. Begin to breathe diaphragmatically. On the next outbreath repeat the number 10. As you exhale, feel the tension drain out in a wave from your head, all the way down the body, and out of the soles of the feet. On each subsequent outbreath, count back one number until you reach 1, continuing to use the outbreath as an opportunity to let go of muscle tension.

3. *Letting go of tension with the outbreath*: muscle tension naturally diminishes on the outbreath as the body lets go to the pull of gravity. Just as in the 10–1 countdown, any breath can be used as an opportunity to let go of tension (from Borysenko *et al.* 1986).

The usual procedure is to teach the patient relaxation during the session and to get him or her to continue this regularly as homework. The exact instructions will vary, but the therapist normally suggests practise once or twice a day for 20 minutes at a time. Patients with sleeping difficulties can try relaxation in bed.

When teaching this technique it is necessary to get feedback from patients about how they are feeling and what they are doing. Summarizing the steps in relaxation before and after teaching the procedure is helpful, and the instructions can be reinforced by giving a hand-out and/or an audiotape. If the session is taped the patient will be able to take away a cassette and use this at home. Alternatively a commercial relaxation tape may be used. Neil Fiore (1984) has produced a relaxation tape especially for people with cancer. If the partner is present he or she can be included in the relaxation exercise.

Once the relaxation response has been learned, the person can practise using it in more stressful situations. They can begin by leaving cues around the house to remind them to relax (e.g. post-it notes on mirrors, the television, etc.) and practise counting back from 5 or 10, allowing themselves to become more relaxed at each step. Once they have practised, people find that they can focus on 'lowering their emotional temperature' by counting backwards and concentrating on relaxing.

Activity scheduling

Cancer can be a demoralizing experience which leads to a progressive reduction in activities. Sometimes this starts when fatigue, nausea, or other symptoms are induced by treatment. Although most people are able to return to a normal life when their course of radiotherapy or chemotherapy ends, some remain stuck in a state of inactivity. Symptoms of anxiety can cause avoidance of social situations; depression produces social withdrawal, loss of motivation, and loss of interest in pleasant activities. A young married woman with local recurrence of breast cancer wanted to leave her job and buy a new house. She and her husband kept saying to themselves that they would wait until she was cured before making any plans for the future. As a result, any possible changes in their lives were met with the response: 'We'll wait and see'. Not only major plans but also short-term plans like decorating the house were put off, and the patient felt a sense of dejection and frustration.

One way of overcoming this inertia is to encourage rewarding activities. For this couple, planning to decorate a room together demonstrated that it was still possible to get on with ordinary life even with the threat of cancer unresolved. Behavioural interventions can foster a fighting spirit and also give the person strategies for positive avoidance. Positive avoidance is the name given to the active, conscious behavioural and cognitive avoidance which allows the patient to concentrate on everyday life without constantly thinking about cancer. The capacity to put cancer out of one's thoughts for least some of the time seems to be a characteristic of many people who are coping well with their illness. Positive avoidance can become a flexible, conscious strategy which gives the patient control over how much time is spent on cancer-related thoughts as opposed to other areas of life.

Information gathering

The therapist finds out when the patient feels low and how this is related to his or her behaviour. For instance, a depressed man might feel most depressed in the evenings when he is watching TV. The negative thoughts associated with this can be identified and activities scheduled which are less passive, e.g. visiting friends. Patient's rate activities for pleasure (P: 0–10) and mastery (M: 0–10) allowing the therapist to see which activities are most antidepressant (see below).

Distraction

By scheduling activities for times when the patient is most preoccupied by anxious or depressive thoughts, he or she can be distracted from them. At times when negative thoughts are very strong, it can be difficult to counter them. Distraction may be the best coping strategy to use until the person's mood improves. Patient, therapist and partner work together to discover the most effective distracting activities, to be used at times during the day when the patient is most vulnerable.

Increasing self-efficacy

Behaviours that give the patient a feeling of control or mastery can be particularly helpful in combating hopeless and helpless feelings. The partner can be a useful informant who knows what gave the patient feelings of success or control.

Increasing motivation

Many people believe motivation comes from inspiration. In the cognitive behavioural model, however, motivation results from seeing the positive effects of behaviour.

The more rewarding an activity is, the more likely we are to engage in it again. The demoralized patient sees no point in doing anything and falls into a self-defeating cycle of inactivity and loss of motivation.

Challenging negative attitudes

Patients who are finding it difficult to cope assume that cancer now rules their lives and they no longer have any control. Engaging in activities that used to be important to the patient demonstrates that life can return to normal. As always, behavioural change can act as a powerful means of achieving cognitive change, through disproving negative beliefs.

Using activity scheduling

Behavioural assignments are a potent component of cognitive behaviour therapy. They can be used as single activities, as in setting the task of writing to an old friend you had lost touch with, or they can be used within the framework of an activity schedule. This can provide a structure for the day or the week. If a patient is too ill to work the week can suddenly look very empty without the familiar framework given by their job. Scheduling in something to do each day, even if very small, can introduce structure to the week and give the person events to look forward to. A weekly activity schedule is often given to the patient at the end of the first session. A blank schedule is reproduced in Appendix III. This is introduced with the rationale which is tailored to the patient's particular problems. Two examples are given below:

Anxious preoccupation

Cancer is such a frightening condition that it takes up much of a person's time in thinking about treatment and what the future holds. Sometimes this means that the rest of life just get squeezed out. Are there things that you are avoiding or no longer doing because of your worries?

Helplessness/hopelessness

You have told me how bleak your future looks to you, and you say you can't see the point in doing anything. We find that many people get stuck in a vicious circle. They give up things because they see no point, and then they get few rewards from life so they become even more depressed and de-motivated. If you would like to try, I think we can break this vicious circle.

As a general principle, when using activity scheduling, it is best to find out when things give patients a sense of control or achievement (mastery) and pleasure. They may find this difficult at first, especially if they are depressed and are not getting any pleasure out of life. Sometimes asking about past behaviours which they might have given up can generate a list, or asking about things the person has always wanted to do. The partner can act as a co-therapist here by reminding the patient about activities which used to be rewarding. The patient's strengths should be used as a guide for planning new activities, and the partner can again be involved in this exercise.

Some examples of mastery experiences might be:

• driving a car for the first time since the operation;

- taking up a new hobby;
- becoming a hospital visitor;
- looking after your grandchildren for the afternoon;
- writing thank you letters to friends who have sent you get well cards.

   Pleasure experiences might include:

- going to the cinema;
- reading a book;
- going on a holiday;
- buying new clothes;
- going out for dinner.

The tasks need to be tailored to the individual's personality. Some people find doing things for others rewarding, others get more out of personal success. In constructing the activity schedule patients grade their experience for mastery and pleasure from 0 to 10. Activities that are rated high on mastery (M) or pleasure (P) can be scheduled more frequently in the next week. Constructing a timetable of the week often reveals blank spaces when the person is vulnerable to negative thoughts and feelings. For instance, an anxious woman found from her record of activities that when her husband was doing night work she would spend a lot of the evening worrying about her cancer. The therapist suggested that she should decide on things she might do when this next happened, e.g. having a book or writing paper by her bed, making a decision to get up and make a cup of tea when she woke up.

   Cognitive distortions can contribute to behavioural deficits. All-or-nothing thinking occurs particularly frequently. Fatigue and depression prevent people from doing things as well as they used to, and many patients will then start thinking that either they must do things as well as before or they won't do them at all. Rating mastery and pleasure can help patients to start grading these experiences, rather than seeing them in black or white terms. Another common distortion is minimization; 'That doesn't count, I was able to do it every day before'. After a course of chemotherapy, it may be a major success just to make a meal. Looking at what the patient is doing provides a means of identifying and challenging such negative thinking.

Graded task assignments

The ability to do things as fast and efficiently as before the onset of cancer can be impaired for several reasons. In early disease physical causes like side-effects of treatment or psychological factors such as depression can affect performance of previously easy tasks. In later disease the effects of pain or fatigue can be debilitating. It can be difficult to adjust to this. The result is often a striving to do everything at the same pace as before the illness or alternatively to give up. We will describe cognitive techniques for dealing with this all-or-nothing thinking in the next chapter. The behavioural concomitant of these is *graded task assignment*. People who are depressed or physically ill cannot be expected to return immediately to previous levels of activity. Tasks can be divided into their component parts and taken a step at a time.

For example, a depressed patient's husband worked out a plan for gradually increasing joint social activities after returning from hospital. Starting with trips to the shops they moved on to increasingly more difficult tasks. Someone recovering from an operation might set themselves the task of gradually increasing their physical exercise on a daily basis, starting with walking around their flat, then moving on to walking in the garden, walking round the block, etc. By breaking down large tasks into small steps each step forward becomes an achievement that can be celebrated, motivating the person to move on to the next task.

Planning for the future

The temporal focus of the patient's daily life can be important in therapy, since the helpless/hopeless patient tends to see the future in an overly pessimistic way. Some patients have very high standards and expect to be able to perform at the same level everyday. This is not possible if they are receiving unpleasant treatments which cause fatigue or nausea, but encouraging patients to match their activity level to their physical strength can overcome this problem. The focus of attention can change to 'one day at a time' and graded tasks can be used to increase activities in a stepwise fashion.

Many patients adopt the opposite attitude to the future. They say: 'I'm just taking one day at a time' and limit their lives as a result. For these people planning ahead is the best strategy. For people who are convinced they will be dead in a month, but really have a life expectancy of years, a 'lifetime goals exercise' may prove a dramatic challenge to their hopelessness (Lakein 1973). Here the therapist asks patients to think about what their goals would be if they knew they could live a normal life span. The aim of this exercise is to extend the patient's timescale and open up ideas about the future. This can then be repeated with the instructions that the patient now knows he or she can live an active life for year—what would be their goals? The final step is to ask the patient to decide what he or she can do in the next week to start the process of moving towards these goals. So, whatever the real prognosis, the patient can now say that significant steps are being taken towards important aims.

The timespan of planning rewarding activities is best decided between partner and patient. Objective knowledge about the disease needs to be taken into account. Some patients can afford to plan years ahead, whereas others might be better off thinking in terms of weeks or months. A statement of intent to go on holiday in a year's time is a powerful stand against the disease.

Behavioural experiments

Many of the interventions in cognitive behaviour therapy are set up as experiments to test the individual's beliefs about themselves, the world, or the future. A behavioural test can prove far more effective in changing negative attitudes than several sessions of discussion. The activity scheduling and task assignments described above can be presented to the patient as experiments. This is in fact true, since neither therapist nor patient definitely knows the outcome beforehand. By examining the thought and its meaning it is possible to devise a specific prediction about what would happen if the person tests his or her negative belief. Behavioural experiments follow five steps:

1 Elicit thought or belief.
2 Make a prediction of what would happen if this belief were correct/incorrect (this should be as specific and operational as possible).
3 Devise an experiment to test this prediction.
4 Carry out the experiment.
5 Evaluate the outcome.

Example 1

Thought: I can't concentrate on anything.

Prediction: I won't be able to find anything I can concentrate on for more than five minutes.

Experiment: 1 Find something which I can concentrate on for five minutes.

2 Increase the time I spend on it by one minute each day.

Outcome: 1 I concentrated on reading the paper for 5 minutes then got so interested I found I had been reading for 15 minutes.

2 I was able to increase the time reading by 5 minutes each day. My concentration isn't as bad as I thought.

Example 2

Thought: Because of my mastectomy my husband doesn't want me sexually.

Prediction: Men will not be interested in women if they don't have attractive breasts.

Experiment: 1 Find out from husband what attracts him to women, e.g. personality, dress, physical appearance.

2 How many of these attributes do you have?

Outcome: My husband values personality and a sense of humour most in a partner. He says he loves and wants me just as much as before. Perhaps he isn't as put off by me as I thought.

Experiments can be set as homework, or they can be done in the session. In both the examples above the experiment could have been done with the therapist present. The first patient could be asked to read something for 5 minutes and report on how easy it was to concentrate. In the second case, the therapist might ask the partner to list all the things he finds attractive about women with the patient present.

Behavioural experiments in the session are of great value in working with patients' anxiety. If a patient is suffering from panic attacks the catastrophic belief about the physical symptoms of anxiety needs to be elicited and then a tested in the session. Feelings of breathlessness can be misinterpreted as signs that the person is going to be unable to breathe and will suffocate. The therapist can get the patient to induce panic feelings by getting the patient to hyperventilate in the session.

Example 3

Thought: When I get breathless it means I'm going to suffocate.

Prediction: 1 If this is really a physical problem, I won't be able to bring it on by simply overbreathing.

                 2 If I don't control my breathing I'll suffocate.

Experiment: Hyperventilate with the therapist in the session. Don't try to control my breathing.

Outcome: 1 The breathing exercise brought on the same symptoms as I get in a panic attack.

                 2 When I didn't try to control my breathing the breathlessness went away more quickly. This is probably anxiety not a problem with my breathing. If I let myself breathe more freely, I'll actually feel better not worse.

Sometimes behavioural experiments do not have the desired result. A depressed patient comes back and reports the homework was a disaster—she phoned her friends as agreed and they were all too busy to see her. The meaning of this for the patient can be examined. What was her interpretation of their responses? Could they really be busy after all? Is she selectively attending to the negative parts of their replies? It may transpire that one of her friends said she was booked up this week but would love to see the patient another time, but she had deleted this from her conclusion. A 'failed' experiment will always give information about the person's thoughts and how they may have inadvertently behaved in a way that prevented the task succeeding. If a genuinely negative response is received to an experiment like this, cognitive work can be done to minimize the meaning of rejection.

The anxiously preoccupied patient

The patient with anxious preoccupation sees cancer as a severe threat which he or she feels unable to control. The future seems horrifyingly uncertain. Uncertainty about prognosis and doubts about whether one has the strength to cope are issues for all people with cancer, but for the anxious patient they assume overwhelming proportions. Behavioural tasks can help both increase control and reduce uncertainty. The following case is an example of how a simple behavioural intervention can effect attitude change.

> Mary was a 56 year-old widow who had been treated for cancer of the cervix in 1984. She received two courses of chemotherapy followed by a radical radiotherapy to the whole pelvis. She then underwent two caesium insertions. The tumour did not respond completely, and recurred six months after treatment. She responded well to a second course of treatment, but although she was free of recurrence she could not free herself of the belief that the cancer was still there.
>
> An analysis of her activities through the week made it clear that she was spending a great deal of time alone with very little contact with other people. The contact she did have was limited to working in her sister's shop from time to time. Although she did this job well she was in constant fear of criticism, frequently thinking to herself; 'They don't

want me here … I'm always in the wrong'. Her thoughts about the illness were most marked when she was alone and feeling bored. These thoughts also became entangled with other automatic thoughts about not being needed. During the session she was able to talk honestly about how part of her believed the doctors when they told her she was free of disease, but when she was alone she was unable to cope with her fears.

The behavioural intervention was aimed at distracting Mary from her cancer-related thoughts when she was not able to deal with them. It was also framed to provide her with more control over areas of her life which she *could* affect. The therapist began by using the weekly activity schedule, and asked her to plan an activity for each day. Activities were chosen which gave her a sense of self-efficacy. She chose decorating her house as one goal which she had been putting off for a long time. Going for walks was another pleasant activity which she wished to pursue. Her self-confidence improved as she successfully painted a room in her house. The positive feedback from these behaviours also began to challenge her beliefs about still having cancer. She said; 'If I was still ill, I wouldn't be able to do the things I've been doing in the last week'.

As the therapy progressed more adventurous tasks were undertaken. Mary began to get involved with a local charity—giving her an area of her life where she could feel needed—and she also started to explore ways in which she could be more assertive. In this case activity scheduling formed only part of the total APT programme.

Mary also attended a relaxation group which gave her self-help skills for dealing with anxiety. As she progressed through therapy she was taught to identify her self-defeating thoughts, and she eventually became able to challenge her beliefs that she was unwanted and a failure.

This use of activity scheduling helps to change the focus from cancer to other areas of the patient's life. For the anxiously preoccupied patient who is concerned about his or her inability to control the disease, this new approach can be introduced in the following way:

'When we see that there is little we can do to exert control in a particular area of our life we feel helpless. This may extend unnecessarily to other areas, where we really do have a lot of control.' The therapist then encourages the patient to look at the advantages and disadvantages of concentrating entirely on the disease. Patients with more advanced disease may find phrases such as: 'You can't have control of your death, but you can control your life' useful in reorienting themselves.

Anxious patients often try vainly to cope with their cancer by desperately seeking more and more information, or trying one alternative cure after another. APT directs and channels their energies with more skilful and adaptive methods of coping. Sometimes it is necessary to put a ban on information-seeking if it is just feeding into a cycle of anxious preoccupation. At other times it is best to help the patient become a more effective information-seeker through rehearsing questions for the doctors or clarifying reasons why particular information is needed.

Another way of promoting personal control is by helping patients to adopt a realistic approach to staying healthy. Doing things to improve prognosis is not confined to the medical treatment of the disease. There are many things that patients can do to promote their own health. These include taking regular exercise where possible, giving up smoking, eating a healthy diet, and finding ways of relaxing. These activities, which are healthy in their own right, may also contribute to the fight against the disease. The patient and partner can make a list together of the things they can do to exert some influence over the disease. This can become a brainstorming exercise, where the couple just put down anything that is even vaguely possible, from vitamin C to aromatherapy. The act of writing ideas down on paper is another step in countering the belief that there is nothing the patient can do. The anxious patient may be using these strategies already, but therapy helps to put their usefulness in perspective. For instance, a woman with ovarian cancer was exhausting herself swimming sixty lengths a session and jogging every day. For her it was necessary to discuss and plan appropriate and moderate use of healthy exercise.

Similar methods can be used to deal with uncertainty about outcome. Behavioural techniques can be used to move the focus away from prognosis of the disease. The therapist can say: 'We cannot do much to reduce the risk of recurrence, but we can help you reduce uncertainty elsewhere in your life'. Activities can be scheduled which are predictable and pleasurable. Engaging in interesting activities also helps to distract from the preoccupation with recurrence. For example, a woman who had repeated worries that the cancer had come back in various parts of her body found that her anxiety lessened over Christmas. The pleasure of looking after her young children kept her from focusing on her disease.

The helpless/hopeless patient

For the patient with a helpless/hopeless response to the disease there is no longer uncertainty and doubt, but a profound pessimism about the future. The person is convinced that nothing can be done to control the disease. Activity scheduling may be even more helpful with these patients than with anxious patients.

> Jenny was a 45-year-old teacher. Cancer of the breast was discovered by her general practitioner and she underwent a local excision of the tumour followed by radiotherapy. After starting radiotherapy she felt depressed, hopeless and angry. She was concerned about stiffness in her arm and feared that she would not be able to carry out her job if she was to receive chemotherapy. She was divorced and had an eight-year-old son. Both her parents were dead and she had very little social support from relatives or friends.
>
> The first target of therapy was a feeling of hopelessness. The therapist explored what goals she might have for the future if she was cured of cancer. This initially proved difficult, partly because of her depressed mood and partly because she regarded any personal goals as selfish. She identified goals which included visiting a friend in France, moving house, doing some creative writing, getting fit, finding appropriate schooling for her son, and engaging in more joint activities with her son. She agreed to try out some of these activities as part of the programme to give her more experiences of success and pleasure and help to structure her time.
>
> At the end of the session the therapist asked for feedback, and Jenny said: 'What's the point in doing these things to cheer myself up if I will be dead soon anyway?' This automatic thought required a cognitive intervention in order to ensure that the homework assignment would be a success. The therapist helped her to consider some of the advantages which might result from improving her mood, regardless of the prognosis of her disease. The rationale for activity scheduling was repeated, and homework framed as an experiment, i.e. let's see what happens if you try some of these things.

Over the next two weeks her hopelessness reduced and she felt less overwhelmed by her negative automatic thoughts. She carried out the tasks she set herself and started to give herself some time during the day, and also began a light exercise programme. Activity scheduling laid the groundwork for more specific cognitive and behavioural interventions over the course of therapy (Table 8.1).

Focusing on the quality of life enhances personal control over the areas of a person's activities that are unrelated to cancer. By encouraging experiences which foster a sense of mastery and control, the therapist helps the person to start interacting with the world in an active way again. The concept of mastery can be explained and the patient asked to make a list of activities which might promote it. The spouse can be involved in this exercise. Another approach is to set up an experiment in which the patient tries out some of these behaviours and rates them according to the degree of control they feel they have when doing them. The activities must be tailored to the individual and, as with all procedures in cognitive behaviour therapy, should be promoted in a collaborative way so that the patient understands the rationale for the experiment, and takes an active part in its construction.

Activities which are associated with feelings of control can vary from doing the laundry to making a model. The patient should be encouraged to set his or her sights realistically. A simple activity like making a cup of tea when done during a course of chemotherapy may be a much harder and more complex activity than when the patient is well.

The partner can be included in all this as much as possible. The relationship should be explored to see if there any interpersonal factors contributing to the feeling of helplessness. Some partners start to do all the work about the house and do not let the person with cancer do anything. If this is the case there needs to be negotiation of a contract where the ill partner can do as much as possible within the confines of the illness. The well partner has to learn to accept as well as to give. This may require specific tasks to be set such as getting the patient to do things for their partner to thank him or her for what he or she is doing.

The helpless patient may report negative cognitions about the extent to which his or her health can be influenced by anyone. Behavioural tasks can be designed to challenge these helpless attitudes. A fighting spirit can be fostered by showing the patient how he or she can actively contribute to recovery.

Following medical advice

This simple strategy is to reframe the locus of control in the doctor–patient relationship. Although the patient may have little say in the choice of particular treatments, he or she does have a choice over whether or not he or she complies with the treatment. Treatment compliance is not a passive phenomenon but is actually an active course which the patient has chosen. Keeping appointments, taking medication regularly and attending for blood tests, are all ways in which the patient acts to increase his or her chances of recovery. Each out-patient appointment represents a conscious choice to work with the doctors in fighting the disease. This can be further emphasized by considering the consequences of not complying with treatment.

Table 8.1 Weekly activity schedule of a helpless/hopeless patient with breast cancer

Time	Monday	Tuesday	Wednesday	Thursday	Friday	Saturday	Sunday
9–10	Travelled to hospital for treatment		Travelled to hospital for treatment	Travelled to hospital for treatment	Travelled to hospital for treatment		
10–11	Travelled home		Travelled home	Travelled home	Travelled home		Laundry.
11–12	Laundry		Post office	Tea and chat with friends	Tea with friends	Shopping	
12–1			Lunch		Lunch at friends house	Listen to tape of therapy session	Travelled to meet sister
1–2			Met a friend for a drink	Lunch and housework		Lunch	
2–3	Gardening	45 minutes writing	Went for a walk	Visit from colleague at work	Shopping	Bought a book	Lunch with sister
3–4	Collected son	Collected son. Drove him to football	Visited next door neighbour	Collected son from school	Collected son from school		Walk
4–5	20 minutes writing. Took son to football lesson	Collected son. Drove him to football	Collected son	Shopping	Collected son from school		Visited friend and sister for tea
5–6	Walked home	Football lesson				Cooking	
6–7	Collected son	Supper	Supper	Supper			Travelled home
7–8	Supper. Put child to bed	Put child to bed	Put child to bed		Supper at friend's house	Supper	Washing up, etc
8–12	Watched news. Exercises	Watched news. Exercises	Watched news. Exercises	News. Phone calls. Exercises	Home	Reading. Exercises	Ironing. Put son to bed

Information seeking

The helpless/hopeless person can be helped to take more control of the illness by being directed to sources of information such as booklets explaining the illness, books by patients, etc. The patient can be encouraged to approach his or her doctor with questions about the disease. The medical consultation is a frightening situation where all the power resides in the doctor, so it may be necessary to work with patients beforehand in order to maximize their chances of asking effective questions and getting appropriate answers. Writing down questions so that they are not forgotten in the out-patients is a simple procedure that may prove useful. Other patients may need to rehearse or role play with the therapist what they want to say to their doctor.

This technique also provides valuable information about the patient's automatic thoughts in the situation. In order to be effective information seekers, patients have to learn to be specific in their questioning. To ease the patient's task, the therapist can inform the doctor that the patient has been encouraged to ask specific questions about treatment. This technique can prove a powerful mastery experience. It also serves to increase confidence in the medical staff, which increases the patient's belief in the doctor's control over the disease. This can be taken one step further by examining the patient's confidence in the doctor and hospital. Where appropriate, cognitive techniques such as reality testing are used to establish the credentials of the therapeutic team with the patient. With a disease like cancer, where a patient may not be able to contribute as much to his health as in other illnesses, it is correspondingly important that there should be trust and effective communication with those treating the patient.

The choice of strategy will depend on the individual patient's problems. As always the therapist needs to be aware of the delicate balance between confronting negative thoughts and feelings about cancer and helping the patient distract him or herself from overwhelming negative thoughts.

Further applications of behavioural techniques

So far we have been considering the use of behavioural techniques to cope with the threat that cancer represents to survival. Concerns about the progression of the disease and life expectancy are often accompanied by concerns about the impact cancer has on key areas of the person's life. In a study of patients with newly diagnosed cancer Harrison *et al.* (1994) found that 50% of patients reported the current illness as a major or moderate concern and 22% were concerned about the future. The effects of treatment (24%), physical symptoms (18%) and inability to do things (18%) also worried people. The distinction between threat to survival and threat to other aspects of the patient's life is often arbitrary in clinical practice. The patient with an anxious preoccupation whom we considered earlier had a chronically low self-esteem. The hopeless patient had also had problems with interpersonal relationships in the past, and saw the side-effects of her treatment for cancer—the stiff arm following radiotherapy—as a sign that she was an invalid. Behavioural techniques can be used with problems arising within these other aspects of the patient's life (treatment, physical disability, relationships, self esteem, etc.).

One patient who had a good adjustment to her disease and did not feel hopeless about the future, nevertheless had depressive symptoms which responded to behavioural interventions.

Betty was a 60-year-old retired office worker with stage III ovarian cancer. She had a successful course of treatment but relapsed three years later. She made a good response to her second course of treatment, but was left with persistent tiredness, early morning wakening and tearfulness. She made a slight improvement on anti-depressant medication from her general practitioner but was still significantly depressed when referred for psychiatric help.

As a consequence of her depressed mood this woman's behavioural repertoire was greatly diminished. She was no longer doing many of the things she had previously enjoyed. This was exacerbated by the fact that she and her husband had moved into a bungalow just before the recurrence of her tumour. A lot of unpacking and decorating was left undone. Her negative automatic thoughts were self-critical—'I shouldn't be like this, I ought to be able to get myself out of it' and 'I'm ashamed of myself for not doing these things about the house'.

She was resentful about moving home—'Everything's gone wrong since I moved' 'I wouldn't have got cancer again if I hadn't moved'.

She was trapping herself by her resentment, because it reduced her motivation to do anything in the new house. But her inactivity led to further negative thoughts about her failure to act like her old self.

Betty was treated with cognitive behaviour therapy in combination with anti-depressant medication. The first week's homework assignment required her to monitor her activities and to start with some small activities—in this case doing half an hour's knitting a day, and clearing three sections of wardrobe as a start to tidying her home. This produced an improvement in her mood in the course of a week. She recorded the amount of mastery she got from each activity and also graded it for pleasure. As is often the case, once she started to get rewards from her behaviour her motivation increased and she did more than she set out to do.

Her mood continued to improve over the next few weeks but her tiredness persisted and she was admitted to hospital a few weeks later with abdominal pains. She was found to be suffering from acute myeloid leukaemia secondary to the treatment she received for her own ovarian cancer and died within a short time.

This case raises some interesting questions. Firstly, was the patient's depression due to incipient leukaemia? Although this cannot be excluded her mood had been low for several weeks prior to the onset of any physical symptoms, and had perhaps been present as much as three months earlier when she was still receiving treatment. Whatever the cause of her depression it responded to psychological treatment within a short period.

Secondly, was it appropriate to treat this lady with APT? If one had known that her life span was so short the particular form of treatment may not have been chosen. However, as is frequently the case, the physical condition of the patient changed during the course of therapy, requiring new considerations and plans. The therapist needs to make judgements on the evidence available from the medical staff treating the patient. In cognitive behaviour therapy problems are formulated as hypotheses. The therapist will usually say: 'Your tiredness and fatigue do not seem to be caused by

Table 8.2 Weekly activity schedule of a depressed patient with ovarian cancer. (Graded activities: M for mastery and P for pleasure)

Time	Monday	Tuesday	Wednesday	Thursday	Friday	Saturday	Sunday
9–10							
10–11							
11–12		Discussed plans for new kitchen units. (M10 P 5)			Knitting 45 min. (M 10 P 5)		
12–1		Knitting 35 min. (M10 P 4)	Ironing 30 min.		Housework 45 min. (M 10 P 5)		
1–2		Tidied section of wardrobe. (M 8 P 3)				Shopping. (M 9 P 5)	
2–3							
3–4			Visited friend. (M 10 P 4)	Went out shopping. (M 10 P 4)			Friend's birthday. (P 6)
4–5							
5–6							
6–7		Visited friend for a meal. (M 10 P 6)				Prepared evening meal. (M 10 P 5)	
7–8				Knitting 35 min. (M 10 P 5)			
8–12			Knitting 35 min. (M 10 P 3)			Knitting 50 min. (P 6)	Knitting 1 hr. (P 6)

any physical symptoms but could well be a sign of depression. Perhaps we can work on your mood and we will see what happens to your tiredness'. This in fact is what happened. Her tiredness improved a little, but did not disappear completely.

Finally, this case example demonstrates the application of graded tasks assignment. The tasks set were at first very simple and undemanding. As her mood improved the therapist helped her to choose more difficult and complex activities. Table 8.2 shows how she gradually increased the time she spent knitting from 35 minutes to one hour over the course of a week.

Summary

Behavioural interventions can provide a very effective means of challenging negative attitudes, providing a sense of personal control and teaching self-help methods. They are usually the strategy of choice at the beginning of cognitive behavioural therapy. Behavioural experiments can be useful at any time through the course of therapy. When setting homework assignments and number of factors should be considered:

1 Tailor the assignment to the individual's needs. Wherever possible, set the task collaboratively and include the partner.

2 Explain, and get feedback on, the rationale for each behavioural task.

3 Make homework tasks as specific and concrete as possible. Write them down for the patient to take away. Make clear predictions about what results are expected.

4 Make the task appropriate for patient's level of education, physical, and psychological ability.

5 Try to see a 'no-lose' situation. When possible make sure the patient will succeed at the task.

6 Ask for feedback on the effects of the task at the next session.

Chapter 9

Cognitive techniques I: basic cognitive techniques

Adjuvant pschological therapy (APT) aims to give patients relief from emotional distress and to change maladaptive adjustment. Cognitive techniques comprise one of the most important sets of treatment strategies in APT, and form an important component of the second phase of therapy. This chapter covers the following topics:

- the application of cognitive techniques, with special reference to the 'Dysfunctional thought record' the most commonly used format for identifying and challenging negative thoughts.

- how to use the thought record to elicit, monitor, and evaluate thoughts and beliefs, and how to devise action plans.

- basic methods for evaluating thoughts and beliefs: reality testing, searching for alternatives, reattribution, decatastrophizing, and weighing advantages and disadvantages.

- further cognitive techniques: distraction, self-instructional training, cognitive rehearsal, and the use of imagery.

- how to work with underlying assumptions and core beliefs.

The application of cognitive techniques

Eliciting automatic thoughts and beliefs

The first step in any cognitive intervention is to identify the thoughts or beliefs relevant to the problem being presented. Once the problem the patient wants to address in the session has been clarified, the therapist starts to explore the thoughts, feelings, behaviours, and physical sensations associated with it (see Fig. 2.3). At this stage it may be helpful to list the patient's experience of the problem under those four headings. So, for a patient worried about fatigue, the relevant features might be

Physical sensations	Thoughts	Feelings	Behaviours
Tiredness	'I can't do anything now.'; 'I'm useless'	Depressed; Hopeless	Withdraw, do less

The cognitive model suggests that the way the person views their fatigue will have a significant impact on how they cope with it. The most reliable method of discovering the meaning of a symptom like this for the individual is through the thoughts he or she reports about it. Reported thoughts (e.g. 'I hate myself') or images (e.g. 'I can see the cancer eating me up') are more valuable than the therapist's interpretations of what the patient might or ought to be feeling. In this context a cognition is defined as: 'either a thought or a visual image that you may not be aware of unless you focus your attention on it'. The thoughts may therefore not be immediately apparent, but may need some practice before the person can identify what is upsetting them.

Beck *et al.* (1979) recommend five steps in teaching the patient to observe and record thoughts:

1 Define automatic thought.
2 Demonstrate the relationship between thoughts and feelings (or behaviour) using specific examples.
3 Demonstrate the presence of cognition from the patient's recent experience.
4 Assign homework to collect thoughts.
5 Review the patient's thought records and provide concrete feedback.

There are several ways in which cognitions can be demonstrated to the patient.

- The patient is asked if he or she had any thoughts about the therapy just prior to the session. Patients may think: 'this won't be of any use', 'I'm not mad, why are they sending me to a psychiatrist?', 'I'm too far gone to be helped', etc.
- The therapist can comment on any change in emotion during the session, e.g. the patient becoming tearful, looking worried, etc. These emotional changes often reveal 'hot cognitions' about the therapist or the therapy, e.g. 'I saw you look at your watch and I thought you weren't interested in what I was saying'.
- The patient is asked to remember the last time he or she experienced a strong emotion. A mental action replay of the situation, step by step, can reveal the thoughts or images that occurred at the time.
- A recent experience can be recreated in the session through role play or imagery, and the patient asked: 'What's going through your mind right now?'

These techniques can be used in any session throughout therapy for eliciting thoughts about crucial events. When eliciting thoughts the therapist should try to establish the various meanings the situation had for the person. As many thoughts as possible should be identified, rather than just stopping at the first one or two, because the first thoughts to be described may be fairly superficial. Asking yourself if you would feel this upset if you thought this way can give a clue to whether the 'hot cognition' has been found. In addition to discussing thoughts in the session, the patient is encouraged to start monitoring thoughts between sessions. When the patient has grasped the concept of automatic thoughts it is vital that he or she starts to notice these thoughts in everyday life, and then find ways of evaluating them.

Monitoring automatic thoughts

Once the patient is familiar with the idea that thoughts are connected with emotional distress the next step is to start recording these thoughts. The patient is given the automatic thought record (Appendix IV) and asked to recall the negative thoughts he or she had together with the situation in which they occurred and the emotion felt. The instructions given will depend on the particular problems. A patient who is depressed might be asked to write down the thoughts every time the depression gets worse. A woman who has an anxious preoccupation with cancer might be asked to recall the thoughts she has every time she starts to worry about a particular bodily symptom. Other patients can write down thoughts on particular themes such as hopelessness or unpredictability. Finally, if the problem is situational, e.g. hospital phobia or conditioned nausea, the patient can monitor thoughts that occur in that particular situation. Specific guidance on what to record and when to do it will increase the likelihood that the homework assignment will be carried out.

In our example of the patient who feels very tired, the homework could be to record times when he or she feels tired (rating the symptom on a 0–10 scale) and then record the thoughts and feelings experienced at the time.

People often need instruction and practice to get the automatic thoughts in a correct form. Useful tips are:

1 *Keep it brief.* 'I'm a failure' rather than 'I was walking home last night and he said something to me which made me feel terrible and it was just like being told I had failed'.

2 Distinguish clearly between situations, emotions and thoughts: The example above mixed them all up.

3 Write statements rather than questions: 'what am I going to do?' becomes 'I can't think of anything I can do to help'.

4 Write automatic thoughts separately, not in a long diary like stream of consciousness.

5 *Make sure you really have got the automatic thought.* Many people put down reality based statements such as 'we're in debt', but leave out the subsequent thoughts which are the ones that are really disturbing, like 'I'm sure they're going to take us to court', 'I can't stand the shame', 'I'm too ill to be able to cope'.

It is best if the patient collects the thoughts at the time they occurred, but this is not always possible. It may be necessary to set aside 15 minutes every night to write them down. When thought monitoring is being set as homework it should be reviewed at the beginning of each session.

At this stage the patient is not being asked to challenge the thoughts. Just recording them is sometimes sufficient to reduce their frequency.

Evaluating automatic thoughts and beliefs

Once the concept of automatic thoughts has been grasped and the person has successfully started recording them, the next step is to challenge them. Because people often describe a lot of thoughts, it is important to help them to find the best thought to challenge. One way of doing this is to take the thought which seems to explain most of

Table 9.1 Automatic thought record of a patient with fatigue

Situation	Fatigue (rate from 0–10)	Emotions (rate from 0–10)	Automatic thoughts	Alternative response	Action plan
My grand daughter came and I felt too tired to play with her	8	Depressed; Hopeless; 10	I can't do anything now. I'm useless	I'm having a difficult time today. I'm more breathless than usual, but I can still play some less tiring games with her. Nobody else thinks I'm useless. I can still enjoy being with her even if we don't play too hard	Plan games I can play in future that aren't too physical. Invite them round on days when I'm feeling less tired
Trying to make the bed	6	Depressed 5	I'll never manage this. I'm useless. What's the point	I did it yesterday, even though I felt very tired. I know that some of this tiredness is psychological, not physical. If I have a go. I'll feel better for at least trying	Don't give up immediately because I feel tired. Try it and see if I can do it

the emotional response i.e. the thought which is most upsetting, and call this the 'hot thought' which the person needs to test. When the thoughts are identified and recorded they can initially be examined for cognitive distortions. Examples are given below.

Automatic thought	Distortion
My husband doesn't make love to me any more. I'm not attractive	Arbitrary inference
No one can love me now I have cancer	Overgeneralization

Finding the distortion can be the first step in demonstrating that the thought is unrealistic. Patients may find a handout describing cognitive distortions helpful at this stage of therapy. One such handout for cancer patients is included at the end of this book (Appendix I). The next step is to complete the alternative response column in the thought record. This is not an easy process, because it involves learning a new way of approaching thoughts and feelings. It is best to complete at least one thought record with the patient before he or she tries to complete one as homework. Some methods for challenging negative thoughts will be described later. In coming up with responses to thoughts on a thought record, the patient must make them personally meaningful. A common mistake is to use weak arguments such as simply saying the opposite of the automatic thought. For instance, a woman with breast cancer might say: 'No one can love me now' (automatic thought); 'People can love me' (rational response). A more effective response might be: 'I know my husband still finds me attractive because he tells me. I'm mixing up love and sexual attractiveness. My children love me, my husband loves me'.

Answers work best if they are specific and based on clearly described and testable occurrences. Table 9.2 summarizes the questions patients can ask themselves when trying to evaluate negative thoughts.

Table 9.2 Questioning negative automatic thoughts

What are my reasons for believing this is true?

What are my reasons for **not** believing this is true?

Are there other ways of looking at this?

Is there an alternative explanation?

What would I say to a friend if they were in this situation?

If it's true is it really as bad as I fear?

What's the **worst** that could happen?

What's the **best** that could happen?

What's **most likely** to happen?

How can I cope with it?

What are the advantages of thinking in this way?

What are the disadvantages?

Devising an action plan

Filling out a thought record is more effective if the outcome is some definite action. If a convincing alternative to the thought is found, this can be used as a flashcard for dealing with the thought in the future. The person can decide to rehearse how to interpret the situation differently when it next comes up. A behavioural task often suggests itself from the exercise. In Table 9.1 the fatigued patient came up with two ways to deal with feeling low because he could not play with his 3-year-old grand-daughter: to think of less physical things they could do together, and to wait until one of the days when he felt less tired and invite her round on that day. Challenging the negative thoughts allows you to be more constructive in your problem solving. In many cases a plan of action becomes obvious from the results of the thought record. If the person is still unsure about whether the negative thought is accurate or not, a behavioural experiment (see Chapter 8) can be arranged to test it. In Table 9.1 the patient determined to try making the bed regularly as an experiment to test whether the tiredness was entirely physical or perhaps a symptom of his depression.

Basic methods for evaluating thoughts and beliefs

The process of monitoring and testing automatic thoughts is basic to cognitive therapy. The techniques the patient uses to challenge thoughts are part of the problem-solving procedure demonstrated in the session. Once the problem is defined, the associated negative emotions are acknowledged and the patient is encouraged to express them openly (see Chapter 7). Then the negative automatic thoughts are elicited and one or more of the cognitive interventions described below is employed to deal with the problem. This is frequently done with the help of a thought record, but on other occasions it may be done through informal discussion.

The techniques described here cover five of the commonest methods for testing thoughts and beliefs:

- reality testing
- searching for alternatives
- reattribution
- decatastrophizing
- weighing advantages and disadvantages.

The distinctions between these different techniques are useful for learning cognitive strategies, but they should not be taken as hard-and-fast categories. As the novice therapist becomes more experienced he or she will find him- or herself using several techniques within a short space of time in order to achieve cognitive change. All therapists develop their own individual techniques which are not necessarily covered here.

Reality testing

Reality testing simply means testing the validity of a thought or belief. The patient is asked to look for the evidence which supports or does not support the belief.

Reality testing is one of the core cognitive procedures. The goal is to distinguish realistic sadness from depression, realistic fear from irrational anxiety. Cancer causes tremendous suffering in its own right, but this suffering may increase when we buy into extreme or unhelpful thinking. Fear of recurrence is a good example of this. Everyone with cancer has to live with a constant possibility that the disease will return. For some people the likelihood of recurrence is relatively low, yet they find it hard not to ruminate about it. Examining the evidence allows the person to form an accurate opinion of how realistic their fears really are. In people with early stage disease and good prognosis reality testing helps to promote a realistically optimistic view of prognosis. Feelings of guilt, self-blame, worthlessness and isolation are also often the result of distorted thinking:

'I will never get a job now that I've had cancer'.
'I'm unattractive'.
'There's nothing I can do about it'.

Skilful questioning draws out the fallacies in the patient's beliefs. In looking for evidence the therapist can draw on a variety of sources:

1 The patient's past experience.
2 The patient's knowledge and observation of other people's behaviour and experience.
3 Reference to reputable sources of information, e.g. books, professionals, etc.
4 Reference to the person's own standards.
5 Rules of everyday logic.

Example 1

Let us take the example of a woman who has recently had a colostomy and is afraid of social gatherings.

Step 1 Elicit automatic thoughts:

'I can't take the chance, I might smell'.

'I won't go, I'm so embarrassed'.

'They'd never want to see me again I'd be so ashamed'.

Step 2 Identify the 'hot thought' that causes most distress:

'I can't take the chance, I might smell'.

Step 3 Look for evidence for and against her belief.

1. *Using past experience*: Has she been to any social events since the operation? Did anything happen to suggest people noticed? If yes, then on what did she base her judgement that someone noticed? (This challenges the distortion of arbitrary inferences.) Are there any alternative explanations for her interpretation that people notice the smell? (Challenging arbitrary inference.) How many people did she talk to who did not notice as opposed to those who did? (Challenging selective abstraction.)

2. *Using knowledge of other people*: Has she asked people close to her if there is a smell? From her knowledge of them are they likely to be lying if they say no? From her knowledge of people, are they really likely to ostracize her if she does smell?

3. *Using information source*: Could she find out from a stoma nurse if this is a problem she is likely to encounter?

4. *Using the patient's own standards*: If she was in a similar situation, would she reject someone because of a post-operative problem?

5. *Using logic*: If she bases her assumptions on the fact she can smell herself, how likely is it that other people can smell her?

These are all approaches that that can be used to test her assumption that there will be dire consequences if she goes to a social event. After working on this with her, the therapist could set up a homework assignment where the patient tested the belief by going into a social situation to find out if people really do notice anything. If the belief did prove to be true, the therapist could help the patient use problem solving to find strategies for reducing the smell e.g. consulting the stoma nurse for advice.

Example 2

This is an excerpt from a therapy session with a 43-year-old woman with breast cancer. On the Hospital Anxiety and Depression Scale (Zigmond and Snaith 1983) she scored: anxiety 19, depression 2. The Mental Adjustment to Cancer Scale (Watson *et al.* 1988) showed a score of 34 (maximum 36) on the anxious preoccupation scale. This picture of predominant anxiety was supported by her clinical state. Cancer represented a considerable threat to her personal domain. She had a strong belief that she could only be happy if she was sexually attractive, and she saw cancer as a threat to her attractiveness. Her doctors suggested that she should be treated with anti-oestrogen therapy, which 'terrorized' her with the thought of having an artificial menopause and ceasing to be desirable. The therapist used questioning to test the validity of her fear.

Patient: When I think of the menopause I think, what unknown terrors are there ahead? ... It's unknown territory.

Therapist: Do you know any people who have been through the menopause and are still attractive?

Patient: Yes, I have one very good friend ... but hers was an artificial menopause ... she's 55.

Therapist: So that would be a menopause similar to the sort you might go through?

Patient: Yes.

Therapist: So you have evidence that it is possible for people to go through the menopause and to come out of it still attractive. Is she someone who still has an active sex life?

Patient: Oh, yes, very much so.

Therapist: And does she say that she's been adversely affected by the menopause?

Patient: No, I mean, I haven't asked her in so many words, but I'm sure not, no.

Therapist: That's interesting because what you're saying is that the menopause conjures up this feeling of terror of the unknown, but your friend's experience
is that it was fairly benign.

Patient: Yes.

This intervention had the specific effect of challenging her belief that there was no
sex life after the menopause. It also had a more general effect of introducing her to the
idea that strongly held beliefs based purely on emotion might be fallacious; the groundwork was laid for her to base beliefs on evidence rather than emotional reasoning.

Searching for alternatives

This technique involves exploring alternative ways of viewing the situation. As such it
can be used as part of reality testing, but can also be used when the thoughts are likely
to be realistic. If the person's negative thoughts are accurate, they may still be unhelpful
and there may be other ways of looking at the situation. People with negative styles of
adjusting to cancer are locked into a mental set which limits their ability see beyond a
narrow range of options. The hopeless patient selectively focuses on the negative
aspects of the future. By asking him or her to list alternative outcomes that might be
possible, the therapist begins to overcome the pervasive negative thinking. At first the
person will only be able to think of negative options, but as the therapist presses for
more alternatives the individual finds that the options become increasingly positive.

The impact of this method can be increased if the patient writes down the ideas in a
list. Putting thoughts on paper allows some distancing, and many people find their
negative thoughts look quite unrealistic when they are written down. This does not
have to be limited to prediction of the future. A useful technique is to ask a patient
and spouse to make a list of alternative ways of viewing themselves. A demoralized
patient will initially come up with a list of weaknesses. The therapist can then say;
'Now let's put down what you see as your strengths, next to your weaknesses'. This
information can then become part of the treatment plan, which should include ways
of building on the strengths of the patient and the partner.

Weaknesses

I worry too much.

I often feel unable to cope.

I rely too much on other people.

Strengths

I care about other people.

Once I make up my mind I stick to it.

I'm conscientious.

I'm reliable.

The weaknesses can also be the focus of attention, firstly to see if the patient is distorting the facts or underselling him- or herself, and secondly, if they appear to be
accurate, they can be put on the agenda as problems to be solved.

The technique can also be applied to finding new ways of looking at cancer. The couple can brainstorm ways in which their lives might be changed for the better as a result of cancer, e.g. spending more time together, learning to take things easy, planning things they always wanted to do, taking more care of their health. If they cannot think of anything then the exercise can be used as an opportunity for encouraging them to plan ways of improving their lives. There is some evidence that patients who can see positive changes in their lives as a result of cancer have a better psychological adjustment (Taylor *et al.* 1984; Tennen and Affleck 1999) and that cognitive behavioural techniques can increase 'benefit-finding' in cancer patients (Antoni *et al.* 2001).

Some changes for the better which patients report include: 'We are closer together as a family', 'We value the time we have together', 'I find simple things more enjoyable', 'We don't argue about trivia', 'Life has more meaning now'.

Another way of looking for alternatives is to ask what you might say to a friend in a similar situation. People who are very hard on themselves over their appearance or functioning are usually much less critical when they look at others. Identifying the double standard can create some leverage in helping the person to view themselves more compassionately. If necessary the therapist can role play an interaction with a friend to reinforce this alternative perspective.

Reattribution

Reattribution is a specific example of the alternatives method. We all try to find causal explanations for things that happen to us. In cancer, it is common for people to try to find someone to blame for their illness, either themselves or another person. A responsibility pie chart can be used to challenge unreasonable blame. For instance a woman who blames herself for her teenage son's bad behaviour might be helped to identify other people and things which might have some involvement in causing and solving the problem. Figure 9.1 shows how the initial response of blaming

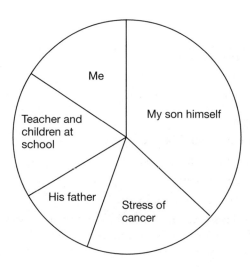

Fig. 9.1 Responsibility pie chart for a woman who blames herself for her son's bad behaviour.

herself 100% was tempered by placing other factors in the responsibility pie. Inevitably the person has to accept that they cannot be totally responsible for anyone else's behaviour.

Bodily symptoms can be another focus of misattributions. Patients with panic attacks tend to focus on the physical symptoms of anxiety, such as palpitations, and interpret them as a heart attack. Reattribution training involves getting them to look at other possible explanations for their experiences. Cancer patients with the anxious preoccupation style of adjustment also focus on minor physical symptoms as signs of a return of the disease. Changing the interpretation of the aches and pains is an important part of helping their anxiety.

Decatastrophizing

The anxious patient will predict the most threatening outcome of any situation, and will have vivid images of the prediction. The person rarely goes beyond this to think in more detail about the real consequences. By continually pursuing the patient with the question: And what would happen next? the therapist can arrive at the most feared consequence. Sometimes the person is able to see that what is feared is not really so bad after all. This process can be repeated in imagery and often the images become progressively more realistic and less frightening.

The same procedure can be used for the more reality-based fears of people with cancer. If the anxious patient fears a recurrence, the most frightening type of recurrence can be rehearsed in imagery. Sometimes the patient can use the relaxation method while doing this. This does not try to make it a pleasant experience, but can help to show the person that it is an experience with which he or she might be able to cope.

A woman who had undergone a mastectomy for breast cancer was told by her doctor that the mammogram performed at a check-up showed some suspicious signs in the other breast, and he needed to repeat the test in three months' time. Although she put on a brave face the patient was obviously very concerned. Exploring her fears allowed her to express her feelings of anger and despair openly. As she cried she was able to identify the thoughts which underlay her fears. These were not directly connected with death, but with the implications of treatment. She thought: 'I won't be able to cope', 'I won't be able to stand it', 'My boyfriend won't want me if I have to have another mastectomy'.

Once she described her thoughts she was able to challenge them very quickly. She remembered that she had coped well before, and felt that she would find it easier now that she knew what was involved. She was also able to see that if this was indeed a recurrence it had been found at an early stage and might not require a mastectomy. Her boyfriend had been very understanding in the past and there was no problem with their sexual relationship, so it did not seem likely that he would suddenly reject her now.

Decatastrophizing did not falsely convince her that there was nothing to worry about. The thought of cancer recurring was frightening and undesirable, but a stress which she and her partner could cope with together. Fortunately her next appointment did not confirm the suspicions and she was given a clean bill of health.

Weighing advantages and disadvantages

A patient was determined that if she had to have chemotherapy she would not go to work and would stay in the house all day. The therapist used questioning to establish what the advantages and disadvantages of this course of action would be:

Advantages	Disadvantages
I would have time to prepare the Bristol diet (but I had three weeks off recently and I didn't do it then)	I'd miss out on lots of things I don't like being alone I would not be getting on with daily life

The benefits and costs of a course of action can be written down and the patient asked to decide if one outweighs the other. As a further step the patient can rate each item for importance. This will give a rough estimate of the extent to which one side outweighs the other. This technique can prove useful when dealing with thoughts about whether to go through with a course of treatment.

Other cognitive techniques

Distraction

Since patients with negative adjustment are plagued with automatic thoughts and selectively attend to negative aspects of the environment, anything that changes the focus of their attention may be of use as an initial coping strategy. Fennell *et al.* (1987) have shown the short-term efficacy of distraction in depression. Simple distraction procedures can be particularly useful with anxious patients. Borkovec and Hennings (1978) showed that attending to pleasant images while practising relaxation reduced subjective anxiety more than did relaxation alone. A person with an anxious preoccupation may be continually monitoring bodily symptoms, e.g. daily breast examination in lumpectomy patients. A vicious circle is set up when non-pathological physical sensations are misinterpreted, causing further anxiety and further compulsive self-examination. This is similar to the selective attention to bodily sensations found in health anxiety (Salkovskis and Warwick 1986). In these cases distraction may be able to break into the spiral of increasing anxiety by interrupting the excessive focus on somatic sensations. Distracting procedures include:

- Focusing on the immediate surroundings and describing them in detail, aloud if possible.

- Engaging someone in conversation—this may help panicky feelings associated with treatment procedures.

- Performing a mental exercise, e.g. mental arithmetic, reciting a poem.

Many of the behavioural techniques used in APT also help patients to distract themselves from negative automatic thoughts. There is always a danger that distraction may become avoidance, so the therapist will ultimately want to help the person address the fear directly to prove it is not as catastrophic as they believe.

Self-instructions

Meichenbaum (1977, 1985) developed the use of self-instructions to facilitate task-performance and as a means of coping with stress. Patients can be taught to prepare things they can say to themselves in times of stress. These should be developed by the patients themselves, and not imposed by the therapist. For instance, a woman with a lung secondary which gives occasional dyspnoea may initially monitor her negative thoughts:

Feeling breathless   →   'I'll never get better.'

Patient and therapist then collaborate to find self-statements that promote a fighting spirit. Whenever she feels breathless she can use this as a cue for positive self-talk, as shown below.

Positive self-statements

'I'm going to beat this.'

'I know the chemotherapy is shrinking my lump.'

'This isn't going to ruin my life.'

'I'm going to get well.'

This form of coping strategy can be expanded to include a whole plan for coping. One patient who was continually troubled by fears of the disease returning developed a four step plan of action:

1 Take a deep breath.
2 Look again (i.e. confront the pain, skin blemish, etc.).
3 Should I be worrying?
4 Reward (i.e. reward herself for coping).

She wrote these instructions down on a piece of card, kept in her purse, so that she could review them whenever she felt under stress. These coping self-statements can be helpful when it is not possible or desirable to complete a full thought record. If a patient has completed several thought records and the same thoughts keep recurring, they can simply put the alternative, more balanced thoughts on a flashcard for easy reference. Not all people are able to use thought records: it is then perfectly acceptable for the therapist and patient to challenge thoughts together in the session and collaborate on the construction of a set of answers to the negative thoughts which the patient can use outside the session.

Cognitive rehearsal

Problem-solving is an important part of therapy and once a solution to a problem has been found, it may be worth rehearsing the new coping strategies in the session. At times this may involve role play but at other times a purely cognitive rehearsal may be appropriate. The patient can rehearse using imagery of the problem and the proposed coping strategy. This technique often produces further automatic thoughts about how the strategy might not work, which can then be addressed. Applications include getting ready for a medical appointment, coping with treatment, etc. The case example described in the section on cognitive interventions for patients with anxious pre-occupation, demonstrates the use of this method to prepare parents for telling their daughter about her mother's diagnosis of cancer.

Imagery techniques

Cognitive rehearsal is only one of the many uses of imagery in cognitive therapy. There are three possible applications to people with cancer: exposure in imagination, imagery modification, and visualization.

Exposure in imagination

Patients who are phobic or who have conditioned anticipatory nausea can imagine the aversive stimulus while relaxed. Although this method is less effective than exposure *in vivo*, it may be necessary when real life exposure is not possible. In the classical systematic desensitization procedure the patient relaxes and imagines increasingly more frightening scenes (a hierarchy of frightening situations is constructed beforehand). Each time patient's become anxious they go back to relaxation until the anxiety is under control.

Image modification

Many images can be identified in people under stress. Depressed cancer patients are more likely to experience intrusive images of past events (often memories of illness, injury or death; Brewin *et al.* 1998). These images are cognitions and as such can be dealt with using the same cognitive techniques we have described for automatic thoughts. Identifying the distortion in the image can help to generate ideas about how the image can be changed. Once the distortion is found the person needs to think of how to modify the image to demonstrate the meaning behind it is untrue. For instance, a woman with a successfully treated sarcoma reported anxiety associated with images of herself as a child. She had been seriously ill at the age of 11 and cancer reactivated memories of herself as a helpless, dependent invalid. In order to remind herself that these were images from the past, not facts about the present or the future, she altered the picture of herself alone in hospital by imagining putting on her clothes and leaving. Images that seem vivid and real can be modified by putting them on a mental television screen and visualizing yourself watching them with a friend or family member. This helps to create distance, puts them in perspective and reinforces the idea that they are mental constructs not perceptions. Unpleasant images can be changed a little at a time until the whole scene is transformed. People differ greatly in the extent to which they can use these procedures, but if images form a significant part of their cognitive content it is worth experimenting with some of these techniques.

Visualization

Some patient's wish to find ways in which they can fight cancer themselves, and may ask about the methods sometimes referred to as visualization. This can be used as part of APT if it seems appropriate for the individual. Simonton *et al.* (1978) and Borysenko *et al.* (1986) give more detailed descriptions of this method.

The patient gets into relaxed state and then conjures up an image of the cancer being destroyed by the treatment and the body's defences. In the image the cancer is composed of weak and ineffectual cells which are destroyed and cleared by the body's white cells. The treatment is visualized as a friendly, helpful image that kills the cancer cells. The images can be whatever the patient chooses, e.g. white cells as the fish eating the cancer, or knights on white horses. At the end of the session the patient gives him- or herself a mental pat on the back for participating in his or her own recovery. This exercise should be practised for 10–15 minutes a day. (Simonton *et al.* recommend three times a day but this may not be practical for most people).

The significant points about imagery (from Simonton *et al.* 1978) are:

- The cancer cells are weak and confused.
- The treatment is strong and powerful.
- The healthy cells have no difficulty in repairing any slight damage the treatment might do.
- The army of white blood cells is vast and overwhelms the cancer cells.
- The white blood cells are aggressive, eager for battle, quick to seek out the cancer cells and destroy them.
- The dead cancer cells are flushed from the body normally and naturally.
- By the end of the imagery, the patient imagines him- or herself healthy and free of cancer.
- The patient sees him- or herself reaching his or her goals in life.

Not all patients take to this method. Many find it frustrating to try to imagine the tumour shrinking when they know it is not changing in size. For some, however, it can be very effective in instilling a sense of control. Visual images of the cancer and its treatment can often be used in other ways, without necessarily incorporating the whole Simonton method. Valuable information is gained by asking for imagery: one patient who dreaded chemotherapy reported seeing a large neon sign which said: *POISON.* Using the visualization method allowed her to reconstrue the treatment as a strong helper—so effectively that she wished to continue chemotherapy even when the medical staff felt it was no longer proving effective. Another patient produced an image of chemotherapy as a monster. This vivid metaphor could be used in therapy, and a number of cognitive techniques were needed to challenge her fears. These approaches must only be used with patients who basically wish to have drug treatment but are fearful of it—trying to convince patients to have chemotherapy against their will is not a function of APT.

Working with underlying assumptions and core beliefs

The emotional problems encountered in oncology are usually less severe and less chronic than those found in general psychiatric practice. APT is carried out over six to twelve sessions with most patients. Therapy cannot afford to spend too much time on past experiences or seek to change fundamental aspects of personality. The cognitive techniques described in this chapter are essentially methods of coping which the patient learns during therapy and applies after therapy has ended. Problem-solving strategies, planning of time, and evaluating negative thoughts can all be used to cope with other life stresses in the future. Within this short-term framework a developmental conceptualization can still prove helpful in guiding therapy, even if core beliefs and conditional beliefs are not targeted directly. For instance, knowing that a patient lost a parent in childhood can alert you to the possibility that beliefs about abandonment and attachment might be important to her, and so help to predict the patient's reactions to therapy. Understanding that witnessing an alcoholic parent has made a person determined never to lose control can help to make sense of their attempts to get total control over their cancer. Sharing this conceptualization with the patient can be very useful. Occasionally, particularly if therapy is continuing up to twelve sessions or longer, it may be appropriate to elicit and challenge the beliefs which predispose to emotional disturbance. This is best done towards the end of therapy when the patient is feeling less distressed: challenging assumptions can form part of the end phase of APT alongside preparations for ending therapy and relapse-prevention work.

Our model of adjustment to cancer suggests that beliefs and attitudes held prior to the development of the disease determine the individual's reactions to it. Attitudes about health and illness will obviously influence the meaning which cancer holds for each person. The interaction between personal beliefs and beliefs about illness is very important in this context (Williams 1997). The commonly held belief that cancer means death is an example of this. Other components of the survival schema may also be associated with underlying assumptions. Some of our patients who have experienced several stressful life events over the years, especially if they get a recurrence of the disease, describe a belief that they just can't win. For instance, a divorced woman of 40 was faced with a recurrence of local breast cancer. Her father died from carcinoma of the liver in 1978, her mother died from carcinoma of the breast in 1979, while her sister died at the age of 15 in a road traffic accident. Over the years she had developed the belief that every time she had felt life was worth living something terrible came along. She had an underlying assumption that: 'If I get too cocky, I will be punished for it'. This interfered with her therapy, because every time she thought about trying pleasant activities or doing something to cheer herself up, she had the thought that something would go wrong. The therapist had to challenge this fatalistic attitude before she could continue with therapy. This is an example of a long-standing belief about personal inability to control events, and it is no surprise that this woman developed a helpless/hopeless response to cancer. Beliefs about certainty and uncertainty will also influence the survival schema. People who believe they must be in control at all times or need to know with absolute certainty and plan their lives in detail will find it difficult to tolerate the uncertainty that cancer brings.

Threats to the self depend upon the idiosyncratic ways people have of viewing themselves. People who have rigid absolute beliefs about themselves in relation to the world may be more likely to react badly if their particular belief is threatened. These beliefs often have a conditional 'if—then' quality to them.

> If something happens to my appearance no one will want me.
> I can only be happy if I can be a successful businessman.
> If I can't look after people, my life is meaningless.

When these 'deeper' assumptions (See Chapter 2) are identified cognitive and behavioural techniques are used to challenge them in exactly the same way that 'surface' cognitions are challenged. Looking at evidence contrary to the belief, weighing advantages and disadvantages, etc. can all play a part in this process. Behavioural experiments can be set out to test the assumption. For instance, a person with the belief that she must look after people to make her life worthwhile could identify the positive and negative consequences of this rule:

Positive consequences	Negative consequences
I'm always needed	I don't get time for myself
I can always keep myself busy	Sometimes I do things because I think people need them doing, not because they really need them
I can feel proud of what I do	My family doesn't get a chance to take responsibility for themselves
I get cross if people aren't grateful	When I can't do things for people (because of my illness) I get depressed

Having established the disadvantages of the assumption, the next step is to create an alternative, more healthy belief, e.g. 'If I respect others and myself, they will grow and I will grow'. The person can then devise new ways of behaving to test whether this new rule applies. Experiments might include refraining from always jumping in to bail her son out when he spends all his money, asking people what they would like rather than acting on her assumption that she knows what they want, and scheduling time for herself. These beliefs are often deeply ingrained and cannot be changed dramatically in short-term therapy. If they are addressed at the end of therapy the patient will hopefully have gained insight into the 'if—then' rules which he or she uses, and also learned strategies to continue the work of challenging these maladaptive rules beyond therapy. Core beliefs are usually not challenged during APT, but these unconditional ideas about the self, the world, and other people can often be discussed openly with patients and strategies devised for future self-help work.

Table 9.3 Cognitive and behavioural techniques

Technique	Implementation
Behavioural techniques	Relaxation; graded task assignment; planning for the future; behavioural experiments
Cognitive coping strategies	Self-instructions; distraction; cognitive rehearsal
Cognitive restructuring:	
Surface	Thought monitoring; identifying cognitive distortions; reality testing; searching for alternatives; decatastrophizing; weighing advantages and disadvantages
Deep	Making explicit underlying fears, assumptions, rules and core beliefs

Summary

The cognitive rationale is explained during the first session, and cognitive techniques are introduced in the second or third session. Simple cognitive techniques can be used as coping strategies, but it is usually necessary to restructure thoughts. Monitoring and challenging negative automatic thoughts is the key procedure and patients are encouraged to carry this out as homework. Towards the end of therapy it may be possible to elicit and challenge the underlying assumptions which predispose to poor adjustment to the disease.

Chapter 10

Cognitive techniques II: applications of cognitive techniques to common problems

In the previous chapter we introduced the basic cognitive techniques and illustrated their use. In this chapter we consider some common cancer related problems and discuss the cognitive interventions that can be used with them. These are:

- cognitive interventions with patients with anxious preoccupation;
- how to deal with fear of recurrence;
- cognitive interventions with helpless/hopeless patients;
- working with anger;
- how to intervene with threats to the self schema.

Cognitive interventions for patients with anxious preoccupation

All the techniques described above can contribute to the management of patients who are preoccupied with their disease. By returning to the concept of the survival schema we can begin to devise intervention strategies. In anxious preoccupation the diagnosis is a major threat, and the person becomes hypervigilant to any potential threat from the disease. Normal physical symptoms are misinterpreted as signs of cancer. The patient feels unable to control the situation and underestimates the coping strategies and rescue factors available. Finally, the objective prognosis is uncertain. The preoccupied patient frantically looks around for ways of controlling the disease and making the future more predictable—seeking reassurance, getting more information, removing all stress, trying alternative treatments. The following case example shows how cognitive techniques were used with an anxious patient. The reader can assess how the cognitive components of the survival schema were addressed during therapy. As an exercise the reader might also note down which cognitive techniques were used.

Mrs W, aged 39, was referred by her medical oncologist who wrote:

> Her main problem is that she is finding it extremely difficult to come to terms with the fact that she has cancer and may die from it. At present she finds she cannot reconcile herself to either of these positions and although I have stressed that we are not in a situation yet where all treatment has failed, it is naturally a realistic fear and I have not tried to hide this fact from her. She herself has requested formal psychological assessment and counselling.

Mrs W noticed a swelling on her neck which was found to be due to a secondary anaplastic carcinoma probably arising from the lung. She and her husband were fully and sensitively informed of the diagnosis by her oncologist. Treatment with adriamycin, cyclophosphamide, and etoposide produced tumour regression but was accompanied by unpleasant side-effects, viz. fatigue, nausea and vomiting, and alopecia. She was referred for psychiatric consultation after she had completed chemotherapy. Her general practitioner had prescribed triazolam for her anxiety, without noticeable effect. Mrs W was an only child of middle-aged parents. She described her childhood as happy. There was no family history or previous personal history of psychiatric illness, but she had always been a rather anxious person with some perfectionist tendencies. She had never had any serious physical illness. Mrs W did reasonably well at school and became a medical laboratory technician, working for 10 years in one hospital. She left her job to get married at the age of 26. Her husband was a stockbroker; they had one daughter aged 12 who had become 'rebellious and difficult' since her mother's illness. The marriage was described by both partners as 'close and happy'. They had many friends and, until her illness, led an active social life. For the last three years she had worked for a charity.

At interview, the patient was found to be moderately depressed and severely anxious. There was no diurnal variation in her mood, nor any evidence of suicidal ideas. She complained that all her usual activities and interests had become overshadowed by constant fear of dying and uncertainty about the future. She felt that she had no control over her life and that she was unable to plan ahead. Her husband confirmed her story, adding that she frequently examined her body for signs of cancer and continually asked for reassurance. She was well motivated for psychological therapy and her husband agreed to participate.

The patient and her husband were seen together for two sessions followed by three sessions with the patient alone. The principal problems identified were:

Pervasive anxiety.
Lack of control over her life with inability to plan ahead.
Preoccupation with recurrence of cancer and dying.
Difficulty in dealing with her rebellious daughter.

It was decided to begin with relaxation training in an attempt to reduce anxiety. This proved unsuccessful. However, the patient rapidly learnt how to identify and challenge negative automatic thoughts. As Mrs W began to challenge her negative thoughts with alternative responses, her husband observed that she was becoming less anxious. The therapist suggested that her anxiety was related to her negative automatic thoughts and therefore could be brought under control by the patient herself. When she found that she could indeed reduce her anxiety by challenging her negative thoughts, she also began to feel more in control which, in turn, further reduced her anxiety. She was then encouraged to plan daily activities which could give her pleasure and a sense of mastery. She began by inviting a friend for coffee, by resuming working and—more difficult—attempting to stop triazolam (Table 10.1).

During the second session, the issue of her daughter's rebellious behaviour was discussed with Mrs W and her husband. It transpired that the daughter's change in behaviour coincided with the commencement of chemotherapy. The parents had not informed their daughter of the diagnosis in order to shield her. The therapist asked the parents to consider the possibility that their daughter's difficult behaviour was a reaction to being kept in the dark about her mother's illness. The advantages and disadvantages of telling their daughter the correct diagnosis were examined. Eventually, Mrs W and her husband decided to tell the daughter the truth; in the remainder of the session, they rehearsed with the therapist precisely what they would say to their daughter. This course

Table 10.1 Record of Mrs W's automatic thoughts

Situation	Emotion	Automatic thoughts	Alternative response
Tidying up	Anxious (50%)	I've been having my period for 2 weeks—what if I have cancer of the ovary? (50%)	It's probably the therapy. Body scans didn't reveal a problem with the ovaries (100%)
Sitting on the sofa—shoulder is hurting	Anxious (60%)	My shoulder is hurting—the tumour hasn't gone (60%)	The tumour has not disappeared completely—**yet**. The pain is much less and I have not taken painkillers for 2 days (100%)
My daughter woke up with a backache	Fear (100%)	What if she has a brain tumour? (70%)	It is most likely she has some kind of virus or that it's psychosomatic (90%)
In bed—trying to relax	Very sad and anxious (70%)	I only believe I will go into remission because I can't face the alternative (my death) (60%)	1. I have every reason to be optimistic because: (a) I feel better and (b) the tumour is responding to treatment 2. I am beginning to accept my mortality

of action had the desired effect: the daughter took the news calmly at first, then became angry because they had lied to her and made her feel excluded, and finally her acting out behaviour ceased as she became more affectionate to her mother.

In the remaining three sessions, Mrs W consolidated the gains she had made. She and her daughter became much closer and her self-esteem rose as she found that her daughter needed her. She returned, part-time, to her previous charity work and began to see friends again. Her anxious preoccupation with cancer receded. There remained the fear of dying. This could now be discussed openly and realistically. The patient faced the prospect that her life span was likely to be considerably reduced. The last negative automatic thoughts (Table 10.1) showed that she was beginning to accept her mortality. Based on the premise that her life would be shortened and that it was vital to make the most of that life, the patient and therapist drew up plans to make her remaining life as rewarding and pleasurable as possible.

At the end of therapy, Mrs W was no longer anxious, she felt in control again and her relationship with her daughter had improved greatly. At four months follow-up it emerged that Mrs W had undergone a course of radiotherapy; her cancer was in a state of remission. Psychologically, she maintained the gains she had made (Table 10.2).

The cognitive techniques described in this example were:

1　Monitoring and challenging automatic thoughts.

2　Reality testing—realistic versus unrealistic fears about the future.

Table 10.2 Case report: Mrs W

Assessment measures	Pre-APT	Post-APT	4 months follow-up
Mental Adjustment to Cancer (MAC) Scale			
Fighting Spirit	40	51	50
Hopelessness	14	7	8
Anxious preoccupation	31	17	18
Fatalism	18	19	20
Hospital Anxiety and Depression Scale (HADS)			
Depression	11	6	6
Anxiety	17	8	9

3 Searching for alternatives (reattribution)—in patient's thought diary.

4 Weighing advantages and disadvantages—over telling daughter.

5 Cognitive rehearsal—of how couple would tell the daughter about the cancer.

The behavioural techniques used included:

1 relaxation;

2 activity scheduling; and

3 planning for the future.

The value of education should not be underestimated. Explanation is a powerful weapon against anxiety symptoms. The therapist can explain how the patient's sensitivity to the possibility of recurrence leads to heightened awareness of bodily sensations, repetitive scanning of the sensations, and misattribution of these to cancer. The patient's own words should be used wherever possible, with examples from his or her own experience.

The concept of a vicious circle of anxiety symptoms can be helpful. Anxiety produces physiological symptoms such as palpitations, sweating, and shakiness. If these are interpreted as signs of physical illness, the patient may think; 'I'm going to die'. This will increase anxiety, causing more physical symptoms and an upward spiral which may result in a panic attack. In other patients, generalized anxiety produces tension which leads to muscular aches. The attribution: 'It must be in my bones', causes more anxiety and tension. The patient now focuses all his or her attention on the physical symptoms, magnifying its sensations and producing further anxiety (Fig.10.1). The therapist can explain to the patient that he or she needs to break this vicious circle in order to feel better. To test whether this information is correct, a behavioural experiment could then be suggested, where the person spends two days attending more closely to the symptoms followed by two days distracting herself, and then decides which method produced less distress and fewer physical symptoms.

Cognitive techniques can also offer help for the patient's fear of being unable to control the situation. The therapist can help the patient look for evidence of how he or

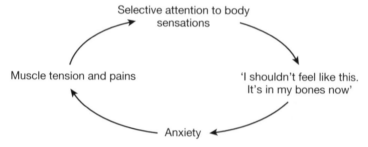

Fig. 10.1 Vicious circle in anxious preoccupation.

she has been control of other areas of life. Here again the focus shifts from cancer to life. The spouse can be brought in to remind the patient of his or her strengths. Similar techniques can be employed for dealing with uncertainty and the fear of recurrence.

Reality testing

How likely is recurrence?

Is the time spent worrying proportional to the risk of the recurrence?

Alternatives

Are there any alternative outcomes?

Why not assume the best prognosis possible with your type of illness?

Decatastrophizing

What's the worst that could happen?

Since fear of recurrence is such a common problem among patients with cancer some scheme for approaching it can help the therapist. We have found this broad plan of use in dealing with people who have difficulty coping with uncertainty about their prognosis.

General strategy for dealing with fear of recurrence

1 Use the best prognosis available from the patient's doctor.

2 Modify the approach according to the prognosis:

  (a) *No sign of active disease*: If the patient is considered disease-free, encourage a search for alternative statements to 'I've got cancer', e.g. 'I had cancer, but all the evidence suggests it's gone'.

  (b) *Active disease*: If treatment might bring about a remission, help the patient to focus on and work towards this. If success is unlikely use cognitive and behavioural coping strategies.

Worry is often a significant problem in people with cancer. In addition to the methods already described for working with anxiety, there are some specific techniques that can be applied to worry. Wells (2000) covers this more fully. Worry may be perpetuated by beliefs about the process of worrying itself. People may have positive beliefs about worry—'If I don't worry the cancer might come back', 'If I don't prepare myself I won't be able to cope'.

And negative beliefs: 'The worry may bring my cancer on again'.

Cognitive techniques can be used to identify and challenge these beliefs. Scheduling worry time for half an hour a day sometimes helps people to put the worries aside until their appointment with themselves. Patients can practise generating positive outcomes rather than their habitual negative outcomes. Finally, many people find the use of a 'worry tree' helpful:

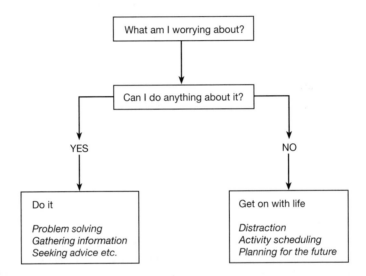

Cognitive interventions for the helpless/hopeless patient

For the helpless/hopeless patient cancer represents loss, and the future is perceived as a bleak certainty. Whereas the anxious patient feels out of control but tries to keep in control, the helpless/hopeless patient, believing the situation to be essentially uncontrollable, has given up. This model can inform the cognitive techniques chosen. The methods used challenge the pessimistic certainty that the future is hopeless. They also help to give the person a sense of personal control. The therapist and patient work collaboratively to establish from the information available how bad the future really is. Evidence for the patient's belief that the future is hopeless is examined, and counterevidence is weighed up. Hope for the future does not rest solely on evidence that there is a chance of a cure. A positive approach to the rest of one's life, no matter how short, can contribute to quality of life.

Many patients think that if they cannot do all that they used to, then it's not worth doing anything. Demonstrating this all-or-nothing thinking is one strategy that can be used with a helpless/hopeless person. The helpless patient is usually seeing the options in a dichotomous way. As if one can either be in total control of the situation or one is totally helpless. Since so much of the fight against cancer is out of your control, you are in a helpless role. The therapist needs to show the patient that with a disease like cancer we can only really work with probabilities and not certainties. In fact, this is not actually different from any other risk in life:

> Never smoking a cigarette reduces your risk of getting lung cancer, but does not reduce it to no risk.
> Wearing seatbelts mean you are less likely to be seriously injured in a road traffic accident but do not guarantee it.

This can be emphasized by getting the patient to rate the degree of control he or she has over various occurrences in life and comparing these with his or her control of cancer. An analogue scale can be used to demonstrate that control on a continuum.

No control [_____] Total control

Searching for alternatives is used to explore things the patient can still do despite cancer. The patient lists activities he or she is still capable of doing. As with all cognitive behaviour therapy, patients are encouraged to monitor and challenge automatic thoughts, but not everyone is able to use the daily record of automatic thoughts fluently. Table 10.3 shows the example of a patient with the salivary tumour who was able to make limited use of the method.

Another woman with her second recurrence of breast cancer felt very sad and hopeless. In the therapy session she was taught to record and challenge her thoughts. The thoughts and responses she produced in the session are recorded in Table 10.4.

Table 10.3 Record of automatic thoughts of a patient with a salivary tumour

Automatic thoughts	Alternative responses
I have cancer—I know I have	The hospital says I have not got cancer
Sometimes I wish this lump in my mouth was cancer so I could get rid of it	You don't because you would not like to go through all that again (i.e. more treatment)
Life is not worth living. I have not changed my life since I've been ill and the cancer will come back	I've got to go on for my family. I can do things to change my life

Table 10.4 Automatic thoughts of a woman with recurring breast cancer

Situation	Emotions	Automatic thoughts	Alternative response
Enjoying a day in the sun	Sad (80%)	I won't be around to see this sun for much longer (90%)	I will be (50%). The doctor says I'm responding to treatment (90%). I've got to be around to look after the kids (90%). I know of a woman who has had cancer in her breast, spine and liver for 15 years. If she can do it I can do it (70%). If I don't enjoy it now it's like giving up (80%)

Working with anger

Some methods for ventilating and channeling anger were described in Chapter 7. Here we present some of the more cognitive and behavioural methods for managing anger. More information on cognitive behavioural methods for managing anger can be found in Burns (1980), Novaco (1976, 1995), Novaco and Chemtob (1998) and Deffenbacher (1999). Outcome studies have shown that the average CBT treated patient is 76 per cent better off than an untreated person with similar anger problems (Beck and Fernandez 1998). These interventions have been studied in people with post traumatic stress disorder (Chemtob *et al.* 1997) but not specifically in cancer patients. Figure 10.2 is a simple model of the processes occurring in people with anger problems. The person with cancer will come to a situation primed with schemas which may make him or her prone to view the situation as an attack or violation. The situation may be directly connected with cancer, and so the unfairness of the person's position is highlighted ('This shouldn't be happening to me'). On other occasions, the trigger may be unrelated to cancer, but because the sense of injustice is present in the person's mind he or she is primed to find injustice in the way they are being treated. So, the underlying resentment about the disease leads to a misinterpretation of events as unfair. Sometimes there may be underlying beliefs about the way people should behave to you if you are ill ('They should treat me more respectfully') which activate the anger. Once the situation is interpreted as an unjust attack or violation of a rule, the emotion of anger is experienced. How the person views these angry feelings will then determine the consequences. If anger is undesirable, dangerous and to be avoided, the person tries to suppress it or over-regulate it. This may lead to breakthrough anger and the other problems associated with emotional suppression described in Chapter 7, and requires intervention to facilitate engagement with feelings and their constructive expression. If the anger is perceived as justified, it may mean that the person does not try to regulate it. This failure of control strategies leads to further anger.

There are three basic steps in the following anger management programme: establishing motivation to change, identifying cues and automatic thoughts, and developing a cognitive behavioural strategy for change.

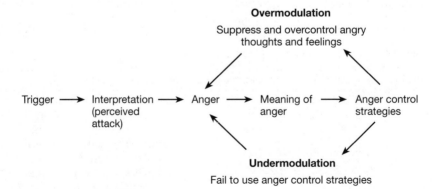

Fig. 10.2 Sequence of events in anger problems.

Establishing motivation to change

It is socially acceptable to think that to have cancer is unjust and unfair. It can also be quite exhilarating to feel righteous indignation, and this is more empowering than feeling a helpless victim. When this anger moves the person to effective problem solving, constructive action to improve services, help other patients, etc. it is healthy and useful. Sometimes, however, anger does not lead to behavioural activation, but may paralyse the patient with impotent rage. At this point it is helpful to explore the benefits and costs of continuing to get so angry. The most useful focus is not on the anger the person feels about the disease but on the anger that is projected or generalized elsewhere. This is not a primary emotion in the sense of a healthy and appropriate response to the disease, but an inappropriate overgeneralization. Distinguishing between the two allows for a therapeutic alliance to be developed with an agreement between patient and therapist to work on controlling the maladaptive anger. Guided discovery is used to show the person how the understandable anger over cancer is spilling over into other areas of life with undesirable effects. The therapist should acknowledge the benefits of feeling angry (not feeling helpless, feeling activated, feeling right) before going on to any challenging, because this will increase the patient's motivation to change and reduce the possibility of a break down in the alliance.

Identifying cues and automatic thoughts

Once the costs of anger have been established (e.g. rows with family, feeling tense, wasting precious energy) information can be gathered about the triggers for angry outbursts. As with any other problem the patient is asked to record angry situations and identify cues for anger. Automatic thoughts are elicited as described above. There is often a sequence which leads (Fig. 10.2) to angry outbursts and it is worth going through the sequence in some detail to establish which actions and thoughts were important in producing the final result.

At the first stage of appraisal one cognitive distortion is very common. 'Should' statements appear again and again in people's thought records.

> 'This shouldn't have happened to me!'
> 'It's not fair, I've been a good person, I shouldn't be treated this way.'
> 'He should be much more considerate!'
> 'He should spend more time with me!'

Although the anger may be directed at God or at fate, excessive anger usually has an impact at an interpersonal level. It is not the railing at fate that causes problems but the snapping at your children. In these situations there is usually a sense of some rule being contravened—'They should have known I was tired.' 'They shouldn't make so much noise.' Gathering information about this is vital before moving on to challenging the distorted thinking.

At the next stage, some people may 'overmodulate' their anger and require emotion-based interventions, whereas others may 'undermodulate' anger. These people may be deficient in the skills most of us use for preventing the escalation of anger: strategies such as standing back from our angry feelings, distracting ourselves by counting to 10, taking a deep breath, talking to ourselves 'Don't go over the top now, it isn't that important', and walking away from the situation. People who get angry under stress may not have learned these strategies, or may be so stressed that they are not using them. This phase of analysing the cues for anger and the person's reaction allows the therapist to ascertain the extent to which the patient uses adaptive or maladaptive coping strategies.

Developing a strategy for change

Once the sequence of actions and thoughts has been established, the therapist can work with the patient to find a weak point in the chain. The cognitive behavioural analysis may reveal a pattern like that in Fig. 10.3. Analysis of the cues for anger can often suggest interventions to reduce the likelihood of anger being provoked—difficult situations can be avoided, or the environment changed to reduce the frequency of their occurrence. In the case shown in Fig. 10.3 establishing a rule that the children must change their shoes before coming into the house might help to reduce the likelihood of the patient's anger being triggered.

Identifying and challenging distorted thinking obviously plays an important part in the anger control techniques of APT. When the anger is interpersonally based, techniques to encourage empathy can be particularly important. The patient may be asked to consider the situation from the other person's perspective. If this is ineffective, more active methods such as role playing the other person in the interaction may produce a shift. Empathy techniques help to show the patient that the person they are angry with is usually not deliberately attacking or hurting them. In the examples cited in Fig. 10.3 the patient might respond to her automatic thoughts by saying:

> My children love me, but when they're excited they can't think ahead. There's no reason why they can't help by washing the floor.
> Only one thing's wrong—the floor is dirty. If I can control my irritability my children are not going to suffer.

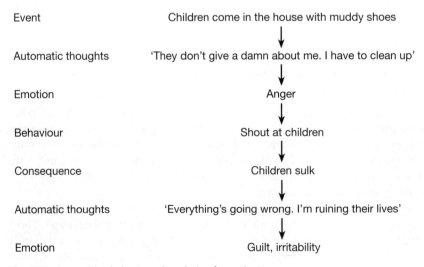

Event	Children come in the house with muddy shoes
Automatic thoughts	'They don't give a damn about me. I have to clean up'
Emotion	Anger
Behaviour	Shout at children
Consequence	Children sulk
Automatic thoughts	'Everything's going wrong. I'm ruining their lives'
Emotion	Guilt, irritability

Fig. 10.3 A cognitive behavioural analysis of a patient's anger.

Once the common thread of 'shoulds' has been identified across angry situations, the patient can monitor their 'shoulds' and replace them with more adaptive interpretations. Following on from this the therapist can look at the advantages and disadvantages of working from a 'should' based belief system and examine the evidence that the world really works according to the rules the patient applies.

Once anger has been activated, the patient can use a number of coping strategies to reduce the affect e.g. calming self-instructions such as 'It's all right, I can handle this without blowing my top', distraction, or relaxation. Therapist and patient may need to work on how the individual can respond assertively without getting angry and this may require role play in the session. The patient can rehearse in role play how to show appropriate anger and achieve his or her goal. Unassertive people sometimes alternate between being passive doormats and having explosions of anger. Patients who suppress anger often fear that when they change they will become nasty people or lose control. Cognitive techniques can be used to test these beliefs, and behavioural experiments set up to find out if saying no or standing up for yourself really lead to the dire consequences predicted by the unassertive person. The therapist helps the patient distinguish between appropriate and useful emotions and behaviours (healthy, constructive anger and assertion) and maladaptive ones (impotent rage and aggressiveness).

Methods for dealing with anger about cancer

Example: 'I've lived a good life. Why should I get this when bad people go scott free?'

1 Encourage direct expression of this anger in the session and to significant others.
2 Find appropriate outlets for the angry feelings.
3 Reality-test the belief that life should be fair.
   (a) Assess evidence that life is fair.
   (b) Look at people the patient knows who have cancer. How many were good and how many bad?
4 Look for alternative ways of viewing the situation, e.g. One patient felt better when she stopped saying: 'Why me?' and started saying: 'Why not me?'
5 Identify the cognitive distortion (tyranny of the 'shoulds').
6 Find the origin of the belief (e.g. in childhood experience or religion) so that it can be reframed as a learned rule not a universal fact.

Cognitive interventions with other problems

The cognitive techniques which one can use to restructure negative self schemata are not very different from those described already. These methods are familiar to practitioners in cognitive therapy to anxiety or depression in the absence of physical illness (Beck 1995; Wells 1997; Persons *et al.* 2001). The therapist must be aware of the meaning of cancer for the individual. Sometimes the person's past experience of illness may be important in understanding his or her reaction to the disease. Someone who has seen a friend lose her hair and become very sick with chemotherapy will be likely to fear the same for herself. The interaction between cancer, other life events and self-esteem may be a complex one. A middle-aged man coped with a serious injury to his wife, followed by his own illness of cancer of the mouth. It was only when he was made redundant from work that he became depressed. The cumulative stress, together with the special meaning of loss of livelihood, constituted the threat to his self-esteem. The subjective threat of cancer to self-esteem is the significant factor.

If we consider again the case of Jenny, described in Chapter 8, we can view cognitive techniques in action. This patient was a divorced teacher with an 8-year-old son. Her response to breast cancer was to feel depressed, hopeless, and angry. We have seen how activity scheduling and goal planning helped her to feel less hopeless in the first phase of therapy (page 95). Cognitive interventions began in the first treatment session and were addressed at her hopeless feelings. The therapist elicited automatic thoughts which confirmed a negative view of herself ('I'm useless', 'I'm handicapped') as well as a negative view of the future ('What's the point of doing anything if the cancer might come back?'). She was interpreting cancer as creating a present and permanent loss from her personal domain. She had lost her ability to function as an independent, normal person, and she did not believe this would ever return. These hopeless thoughts had to be dealt with before the behavioural homework was set. In the next session she was asked to start recording her thoughts, and the concept of reality testing was explained to her. She took well to the task of monitoring and challenging negative automatic thoughts (Table 10.5).

She was due to receive a course of adjuvant chemotherapy, but was very concerned about the possible side-effects. She described how she felt that just as she was beginning

Table 10.5 Jenny: recording and evaluating negative automatic thoughts

Situation	Emotions	Automatic thoughts	Alternative response
Thinking about friends	Alone; depressed	My life has become a nightmare. It's out of my control	If I make a conscious effort I can maintain some control
In the kitchen	Despondent	Once the chemotherapy gets going there are lots of things I won't want to eat and I'll start losing weight again	I can buy convenience foods because its probably the effort of preparing the foods that's the problem
Working at something	Anxious	I've only got a fraction of the energy I used to have and that could be permanent	I may be depressed. Even if I feel tired its better to stay active because I will achieve more
Getting up in the morning	Sad	There are so many things I haven't done and will never do	People do different things in life and mine hasn't been so bad. I could make an effort to do what I want to do

to do more and feel more in control of her life, she would be tired and ill as a result of the treatment. The therapist helped her to test this automatic thought by questioning her about the evidence that chemotherapy had to be so toxic. In fact she had already had a short course of chemotherapy before starting radiotherapy and had not felt significantly unwell. The therapist then went on to ask about the advantages and disadvantages to her of receiving treatment. Jenny came up with the following list:

Advantages	Disadvantages
I won't have regrets and worries	I will lose weight
I may have a statistical advantage and live longer	I will be tired and find everything difficult
	I won't be able to talk to people without feeling sick
I will be able to look after my son for longer	I will become sterile

This procedure helped her to put her ideas about chemotherapy into perspective. Here is Jenny's own account of the cognitive techniques she learned to use in therapy.

When I stopped having overwhelming negative thoughts but went on monitoring what I was thinking, I was surprised to discover that a great number of my thoughts were negative in one way or another and that I seem to have a bottomless fund of them. Negative thoughts seemed to hang together like a string of sausages, and I gradually found that it was a good idea to try to snip them off. I understood what the therapist was saying about thoughts containing distortions … and I found that sometimes I could deal with my thoughts in a different way, taking account of the fact that they could contain a lot of mistakes and noticing when a train of thought was leading to no good.

Chapter 11

Working with couples

The problems of living with cancer affect not only the patient but also the immediate family, particularly the spouse or partner. Yet until fairly recently the emotional distress experienced by the partner has received scant attention in the literature. It seems as if the patient's problems have almost completely overshadowed those of the partner. In this respect, the literature reflects what is commonly observed in clinical practice, viz. that, because they do not have cancer themselves, the partners deny or minimize their own distress and feel guilty about expressing it, let alone seeking help. The few systematic studies which have been published confirm the clinical impression of undisclosed psychological morbidity in spouses and partners of cancer patients (e.g. Lichtman and Taylor 1986; Moynihan 1987). Similar factors seem to predict morbidity in both patients and partners (lack of social support, uncertainty, hopelessness and distress over symptoms; Northouse *et al.* 1996). Psychological disturbance in the partner has a detrimental effect on the patient. Not surprisingly, the quality of the relationship also influences the patient's well-being. Partners who have a more affiliative relationship (Fuller and Swenson 1993) or who are actively helpful (Pistrang and Barker 1995) assist in promoting well-being. Hence, the main purpose of including the spouse in APT is to ameliorate psychological distress in both partners. This can be achieved primarily by enhancing the quality of the relationship between partners. When the relationship is already strong, the partner can act as a 'co-therapist', helping particularly with cognitive and behavioural assignments outside the session.

Not all patients wish their spouses to be included in therapy; some people prefer to explore their feelings and cancer-related problems alone with the therapist. Clearly, the patient's wishes are paramount. During the first APT session, the possibility of including the spouse or partner is raised with the patient and, if the patient agrees, the spouse is invited to take part in subsequent sessions. We adopt a flexible approach, enabling the patient and spouse to decide how many joint sessions they wish to have. In this chapter we present:

+ how to facilitate open communication between patient and partner;
+ the nature of relationship schemas in cancer;
+ basic cognitive techniques for working with couples;
+ examples of couples problems and how to deal with them;
+ ways to engage the partner as a co-therapist;
+ methods for treating sexual dysfunction.

Encouraging open communication

In most cases, marriages are not impaired by the experience of cancer; indeed, some marriages actually improve as the trauma of cancer brings the patient and spouse closer together (Morris *et al.* 1977; Hughes 1987; Zucchero 1998). But as discussed in Chapter 1, there is evidence of deterioration of marital relationships in a substantial minority of patients. A common cause of such deterioration is lack of communication between the patient and spouse or partner (Lichtman and Taylor 1986). In a study of couples where the woman was newly diagnosed with breast cancer, Hilton (1994) identified three main patterns of discussion about fears and doubts. In the first the couple were in agreement that talking openly was the best policy, in the second couples agreed not to discuss the illness with each other, and in the third the two partners held differing views about talking openly about their feelings. It was this last group which demonstrated more problems in their communication. Selective open disclosure was perceived as the most satisfactory of the patterns. Some barriers to communication have been described by Wortman and Dunkel-Schetter (1979). Patients and spouses often adopt a cheerful facade which belies the way they feel. The responses of spouses are determined by feelings of fear about cancer and the belief that they must appear cheerful and optimistic. As a result, the spouse may show discrepancies between word and deed, encouraging the patient verbally while at the same time avoiding any discussion about cancer or even avoiding the patient. The effect on the patient is likely to be a sense of rejection and loss of self-esteem. In order to regain the spouse's sympathy and love, the patient may then attempt to suppress all negative feelings associated with cancer.

Encouraging expression of thoughts and feelings about cancer

In order to overcome these barriers to communication, it is essential to encourage each partner to express freely all feelings including anger, fear, and sadness. The techniques described in Chapter 7 can be used to facilitate emotional expression. We usually begin by asking the person with cancer to talk about how he or she feels. Having learned how the patient really feels, the spouse is then encouraged in the same way to express feelings openly. The patient is often surprised to find that behind the spouse's cheerful façade there is anxious concern and sadness. This discovery can be a proof to the patient of how much the spouse cares. Moreover, it may make the patient feel less helpless and more in control, since the patient can now do something to help and comfort the spouse.

Listening and empathic communication

When the therapist initiates emotional communication in this way it usually allows the couple to share their doubts and fears constructively. If they communicated effectively in the past, the obstacles set up by cancer may be broken down, and they can go on to talk about their feelings together outside the session. Some couples, however, may not have been very good at talking even before the illness struck. In this case, both partners need to practise listening as well as expressing their feelings within the therapy session. Signs that more work needs to be done on communication training include:

- One partner interrupts or talks over the other e.g. because they have difficulty tolerating strong emotions or because they need to control their partner.
- One partner tells the other what he or she is feeling (Mind reading).
- Expression of feelings involves recrimination or blame of the other partner.
- Both partners talk together.

The therapist asks the couple to take it in turns to describe their thoughts and feelings to each other. The partner who is listening is instructed to ask questions so that they get as clear an understanding as possible of what their partner is experiencing (tuning in to their wavelength). They are shown how to reflect empathically back through non-verbal gestures, through repeating and paraphrasing the partners words (thought empathy) and through feeding back what they understand of their partner's feelings (feeling empathy). The therapist may initially need to model how to listen and reflect, and then allow the couple to try this out. The partner who has been expressing their feelings can then give feedback on whether or not he or she felt heard and understood. After the feedback the exercise can be repeated.

Communication training of this kind can be particularly helpful for the spouse of the cancer patient who may be tempted to control, undermine, or invalidate the patient's experience, often for the best possible reasons. Simonton *et al.* (1978) state that: 'the single most important thing the family can offer is the willingness to go through this experience with the patient'. One danger is responding by making the patient too dependent.

Patient: I'm afraid of the treatment. I really don't want it. I don't think it will help me.

Babying reply: Now, you know you've got to take it. It won't hurt you. It's good for you. And that's all we going to hear about it.

Simonton *et al.* suggest an alternative reply:

Supportive reply: I know how you feel. The treatment scares me too and I don't really understand all that's involved. But we're in this together and I'll go through it with you and help as much as I can.

Patient and partner may need to allocate time to talk and practise listening in this way as a homework assignment.

Cognitive techniques

Relationship schemas

As we have discussed in previous chapters, we all bring certain assumptions and expectations to relationships, which are derived from our past experience. We have tacit rules about the way families behave which we learn from our own families as children. These usually reflect cultural and social norms, but each family has its own idiosyncratic rule system as well. Cultural stereotypes include beliefs like: 'A woman's place is in the home'. Idiosyncratic family rules are much more variable, e.g. 'Parents should do everything they possibly can for their children at all times' or 'Parents should expect their children to do things for themselves or they will never stand on their own two feet'. These rules are rarely discussed. They are expectations about how things ought to be. One of the most important sets of beliefs is about illness and how the family should respond to it (Williams 1997). If the patient and spouse hold different beliefs this can lead to difficulties. These beliefs often involve assumptions about how the cancer patient and family members should think, feel, and behave.

Differing assumptions about attitudes to cancer

You should *always* think positively.	You should expect to feel sad all the time if you have cancer.

Differing assumptions about emotional expression

It's better not to talk about your feelings.	You should let your feelings out as much as possible.
Expressing feelings is a sign of weakness.	Expressing negative emotions is natural.

Differing assumptions about illness-related behaviour

When you are ill you should let the family take over for you.	I have to be a perfect mother even if I am ill.
If I get back to work too quickly, I might bring the cancer back.	Everything has to return to normal as soon as possible.

If family members do not express these beliefs they will assume that others in the family are using the same rules. They then misinterpret each others behaviour making inaccurate attributions about people's motives. For instance, if the partner of a woman with cancer believes it is weak to express strong feelings, he may not indicate how upset he is by what has happened. She in turn may interpret his stoicism as a sign that he doesn't care. Case examples 1 and 2 below demonstrate how misinterpretations and invalid assumptions can lead to marital difficulties.

When the quality of a relationship has been poor for some time, maladaptive beliefs and behaviours become solidified. Attributions about the causes of the partner's behaviour become global and generalized. Failing to remember something is ascribed to stupidity, an irritable outburst is put down to bloody mindedness, feeling too tired to do the housework is a sign of laziness. These rigid schemas form a template which leads the couple to look out constantly for information which confirms their negative views of each other and ignore information which does not fit with the schema. Examples 3 and 4 show how negative schemas created very skewed picture of partners' behaviour.

Challenging misinterpretations

Conducting a cognitive behavioural analysis of the couple's problem interaction(s) is the first step. The therapist asks each partner separately for their view of the interaction, what they thought, what they did, what their partner did, and what this meant to them. The interaction can be drawn out on a piece of paper or on a whiteboard.

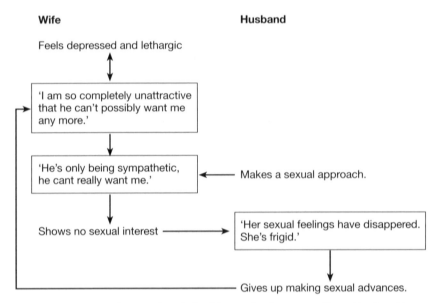

Fig. 11.1 Cognitive behavioural analysis of interaction between wife and husband in case example 1.

Example 1

After a mastectomy a young woman lost interest in sex. She felt depressed and lethargic. Her negative thoughts centred on her disturbed body image: 'I am so completely unattractive that he can't possibly want me any more'. When her husband made a sexual approach she rebuffed him, thinking: 'He's only being sympathetic, he can't really want me'. Unaware of her automatic thoughts her husband became prey to thoughts of his own: 'Her sexual feelings have disappeared. She's frigid'. He gave up making sexual advances.

Simply drawing this diagram may be sufficient to allow the couple to correct their misperceptions. If further work is needed the next step might be to identify the cognitive distortions involved. Example 1 demonstrates the common cognitive distortion of *arbitrary inference*. The partners assume that they understand the motives behind each other's actions but get it wrong. This 'mind-reading' bias can be discussed with the couple, and the disadvantages of jumping to conclusions identified.

In some cases it may be necessary to use cognitive techniques to evaluate the couple's thoughts and beliefs. All of the standard methods of reality testing, searching for alternatives, etc. (Chapter 9) can be applied. When interpersonal rules are uncovered, the costs and benefits of living by these rules can be explored.

Example 2

A woman with cancer had always been the dominant partner in the relationship. The husband was a banker who worked very hard. He would come home after a day at work expecting his dinner. He found it difficult to cope with his wife's dependence, while she felt rejected by his anger. Both partners were using characteristic cognitive distortions.

Husband: If you're not in hospital any more you must be well (all-or-nothing thinking)
Patient: He doesn't love me any more (arbitrary inference)

After helping the couple to reconstrue the situation, the therapist ends by developing an action plan with them. What can they now go on to do with this new knowledge? The couple in Example 1 might decide to spend some time together cuddling and showing affection without engaging in sexual activity to show each other they still care about each other. Approaching intimacy in this non-threatening way could allow them to re-establish trust and so move on to re-establishing their sexual relationship. The couple in Example 2 might agree to a compromise, where the wife does more as a way of showing her husband she is active in her recovery, but he does more to look after her, acknowledging that he cares and that she is not yet completely well. When setting up behavioural assignments, therapists often use the principle of 'give to get'. When couples are resentful of each other it may be difficult to concede to the other partner, so setting up a contract where each agrees to do something for the other can feel more just. If there are two opposing positions as in Example 2, the middle ground may allow both partners to feel they are getting something out of the exchange.

In Examples 3 and 4 we describe some ways of working with more entrenched relationship schemas.

Example 3

A young woman had unresponsive breast cancer. Her husband had sprained his ankle the day before. He asked her to take him to the shops to get some cigarettes. She thought: 'Why can't he go himself? He takes me for granted'. Rather than being honest, she retorted by saying: 'I'm not getting dressed yet, I may wait till this afternoon'. This caused her husband to escalate his demands and eventually force her to take him. It emerged that both partners had schemata concerning the other taking them for granted, and feeling unsupported. Therapy consisted of demonstrating the schema, and encouraging more thought about what the other's perception of the situation may be. The other part of therapy with this couple involved finding more adaptive ways of expressing their feelings of being mistreated, without using emotive language which inevitably upset the spouse.

The final intervention with this couple can be done on a behavioural level. The patient was constantly talking of cancer and admitted she had little time for anything else. The interactions in the relationship had become negative. Simply getting both partners to say what they like and then promoting an interchange of positive behaviours may help to improve the relationship.

Example 4

A woman with carcinoma of the cervix was being treated with APT for problems with anxiety. Early in therapy it became clear that she had a negative schema concerning her husband whom she perceived as old, boring, and possessive (she was 50 and he was 60). This global negative view was so strong that she interpreted all his attempts to support her in a very idiosyncratic way. He was keen to look after her and make sure she did not over exert herself—but she thought, showed that he treated her 'like a geriatric', because, being old, he wanted a 'geriatric wife'. When he asked her how she was feeling, she saw this as evidence that he actually wanted to keep her ill and dependent. The pervasive negative schema caused her to distort all the evidence concerning her husband's behaviour.

Therapy tried to focus on the marital problem, and in joint sessions evidence accumulated that he was indeed concerned about his wife and frightened. She would not change her beliefs at all, which seemed to have been in existence long before the cancer, and APT was not successful. This raises questions about the effectiveness of APT when marital problems are deeply entrenched. In retrospect, it might have been better to work with this woman individually, concentrating solely on her individual coping strategies.

Spouse/partner as co-therapist

Work on communication and cognitive restructuring is not required with all couples. If the relationship is good and the partner supportive, he or she can be a helpful presence in the session and even act as a co-therapist. There are a number of ways in which the spouse can make a valuable contribution:

1 Allowing the patient to express negative feelings in an atmosphere of acceptance.
2 Participating in self-help assignments.
3 Helping the patient to make decisions.
4 Providing practical support when required.
5 Encouraging and participating in joint activities.
6 Helping the patient to regain self-esteem and control over his or her life by encouraging him or her to carry out those tasks and activities which are within his or her and reach.
7 Adopting a positive attitude towards outcome.
8 Providing information on past strengths, interests, and positive experiences which the patient may not be able to easily recall.

Treatment of sexual difficulties

There is documented evidence of impaired sexual functioning in a substantial proportion of patients with cancers of the breast (Morris *et al.* 1977; Maguire *et al.* 1978), bowel (Devlin *et al.* 1971; Williams and Johnston 1983), female genital tract (Anderson 1986; Cochrane *et al.* 1987), prostate (von Eschenbach 1986) and testis (Rieker *et al.* 1985; Moynihan 1987). The main causes of sexual dysfunction are not mutually exclusive. They are:

◆ Loss of self-esteem resulting from disfiguring surgery (e.g. colostomy, mastectomy) or feelings of being 'unclean' or contagious due to cancer.
◆ Physical effects of the disease (e.g. pain, bleeding, weight-loss) and of cancer treatments (e.g. nerve damage in abdominoperineal resection), or fatigue, nausea, hormonal changes induced by chemotherapy and radiotherapy.
◆ Cancer related psychological disorders such as depression, feelings of helplessness, anxious preoccupation with the disease and its recurrence.
◆ Lack of communication between the patient and partner (as described earlier).
◆ Pre-existing marital or sexual difficulties.

Treatment of sexual dysfunction in the context of APT can be outlined as follows. A sexual history should be obtained from the patient and spouse as part of the medical/psychiatric history. It is important to inquire about sexual adjustment as most patients will not reveal problems in this area unless specifically asked. Having established the presence of sexual dysfunction, the next question is whether such dysfunction is causing distress to the patient or spouse. In our experience and that of other workers (Andersen 1986), impairment of sexual function is not necessarily a source of distress to patients. Clearly, it is only in those cases where sexual dysfunction causes problems that therapy is indicated.

Therapy for sexual difficulties is based on cognitive and behavioural methods. Crucial to sex therapy is the encouragement of open communication and expression of feelings between the patient and partner, as described earlier. Accurate information is provided to correct misapprehensions and to allay any fears, for example, that intercourse can lead to recurrence of cancer. In this way, negative expectations about making love can be countered. Resumption of love-making as soon as is desired and medically feasible is encouraged. If intercourse is not possible for medical reasons, cognitive restructuring is useful; ways of re-establishing physical closeness, of pleasing each other sexually without intercourse can be explored. Finally, for some sexual disorders such as psychogenic impotence or vaginismus, Masters and Johnson's (1970) behavioural techniques are appropriate.

Case Example: Illustrating how working with couples is integrated into the course of APT

A was a 32-year-old man who developed a painful swelling of his left testis. A seminoma (Stage 1—early disease) was diagnosed and an orchidectomy performed, followed by a course of radiotherapy. Despite being given an excellent prognosis, he became increasingly depressed and was referred for psychiatric consultation two months after competing radiotherapy.

He had had a normal childhood, and had one brother who was treated successfully for a seminoma. There was no family or personal history of psychiatric illness. The patient had worked for 10 years as a car spray-painter. He had been married for eight years and had one son aged five. The marriage was described as reasonably happy until a few months before referral, when A's withdrawal and taciturn behaviour led to considerable estrangement. His wife described A's premorbid personality as sensible, well-balanced, and fairly passive.

On a psychiatric examination he gave a history of four months' increasing depression, listlessness, apathy, loss of libido, loss of interest, and insomnia. He felt unable to return to work. He showed some motor retardation, spoke in a low monotone and was clearly depressed. He admitted to some suicidal ideas. A diagnosis of depressive illness was made and fluvoxamine 100 mg *noct* prescribed. Because of side-effects, however, the patient stopped this drug after only two doses.

The patient was seen alone for the first session and together with his wife for five further sessions. During APT, the automatic thoughts of the patient and his wife were elicited; they were taught to challenge these thoughts and to keep a daily record.

Example (A) *Automatic thought*: I'm not the same anymore because of the cancer so I won't be able to go back to work.

Rational response: My fear of returning to work came from my *feelings* about myself since I got cancer, not from the disease itself. I have been told that I don't have any sign of cancer now and that my chances are very good.

Example (A's wife) *Automatic thought*: He's changed completely since he was in hospital. This cancer business has made him withdraw completely and, to be honest, I think he has stopped loving me.

Rational response: Being told that he had cancer and having a testicle removed must have been an awful shock. It takes time to get over this.

The patient was urged to plan his daily activities and, in particular, to engage in those activities which would provide pleasure or a sense of achievement. Considerable collaborative effort was devoted to finding the patient's strengths and building on these. For example, after initial resistance, when he protested that he was unable to do anything at all, he was persuaded to take his son out to play football and to decorate the bathroom. He found that these activities raised his self-esteem and were pleasurable. As a result, his mood began to lift; his wife reported that he was whistling in the bathroom, something he had not done for several months.

Communication between A and his wife was facilitated during joint sessions. Mrs A was able to tell him that she had become depressed as well as angry because he had withdrawn from her and, seemingly, given up. Before therapy, she had been unable to let him know her feelings because, in view of his cancer, she felt she had no right to complain. She had, however, expected him to know how she felt without having to tell him (Beck's arbitrary inference). The patient, in fact had no idea.

Another issue that emerged was that the patient regarded his wife as excessively dominant and thought this was her nature and therefore unalterable. Mrs A on the other hand did not wish to be dominant but felt that she had been compelled to adopt this role by his unwillingness to make decisions ('he always leaves everything to me'). Through frank communication, A and his wife came to recognize and learn to overcome these problems.

The patient's lack of assertiveness had caused difficulties not only in his marriage but at work for several years; he had felt angry because there were no precautions taken against inhaling paint spray. A had never expressed his concern and anger, fearing that he might lose his temper and get the sack.

During APT, we rehearsed how he could express his concern appropriately to his foreman. He returned to work after five months' absence, just before completing APT. He managed to speak to the foreman and insist politely on the need for facemasks to be provided. As a result the patient's self-esteem rose markedly.

Tables 11.1 and 11.2 shows the effects of APT on Hospital Anxiety and Depression (HAD), Mental Adjustment to Cancer (MAC), and the Psychosocial Adjustment to Illness Scale (PAIS) scores obtained by the patient and his wife. It is clear from Table 11.1 that the patient's anxiety and depression improved markedly, that he became less helpless, that he lost most of his symptoms (as measured on the Rotterdam Symptom Checklist) and that his psychosocial adjustment (as measured by the PAIS—with lower scores indicating better adjustment) had improved. His wife's depression improved but her anxiety remained much the same (Table 11.2); there was a slight improvement in her psychosocial adjustment. The improvement observed in both partners after six APT sessions was maintained during the following months.

Table 11.1 APT assessments of patient A

	Pre-therapy	Post-therapy	4-months post-therapy
Hospital Anxiety and Depression (HAD) Scale			
Depression	8	0	2
Anxiety	7	1	5
Mental Adjustment to Cancer (MAC) Scale			
Fighting spirit	44	51	52
Helplessness	13	6	7
Anxious preoccupation	21	21	17
Fatalism	17	16	14
Rotterdam Symptom Checklist	19	5	4
Psychosocial Adjustment to Illness Scale (PAIS)			
Total score	58	37	40

HAD scale: Zigmond and Snaith (1983); MAC scale: Watson *et al.* (1988); Rotterdam Symptom Checklist: de Haes *et al.* (1987); PAIS: Derogatis (1983).

Table 11.2 APT assessments of patient A's wife

	Pre-therapy	Post-therapy	4-months post-therapy
Hospital Anxiety and Depression (HAD) Scale			
Depression	7	2	2
Anxiety	10	7	8
PAIS—Total score	52	46	44

HAD scale: Zigmond and Snaith (1983).

Summary

With the patients' agreement and where circumstances permit, the spouse or partner should be included in APT. Joint sessions should include some or all of the following tasks:

- Encouraging open expression of feelings.
- Facilitating communication between the partners.
- Identifying maladaptive interactions.
- Identifying cognitive distortions and challenging automatic thoughts.
- Encouraging mutually rewarding behaviours.
- Treating sexual dysfunction where appropriate.

Chapter 12

Advanced and terminal illness

APT was first developed for the treatment of early cancer, where the possibility of cure allows a strong fighting spirit to be inculcated. However, it can also be used in the later stages of the disease. Throughout this book we have tried to demonstrate how cognitive behavioural techniques can help a broad spectrum of patients with different types of cancer and different life expectancies. In this chapter we consider some of the special issues that arise when treating patients with advanced disease.

In early cancer, treatments may bring hope of lasting remission or cure, and following this there may be substantial disease-free periods. Psychological problems in this phase respond well to cognitive behaviour therapy. The negative thoughts experienced are often clearly distorted and evidence is available to challenge them. Patients may have unrealistic beliefs about the effectiveness of treatment, the impact of side-effects on their lives or their ability to cope. Identifying and testing these beliefs by accessing appropriate information or setting up behavioural experiments is usually very helpful. Once the initial shock of diagnosis is over, it is not too difficult to promote a fighting spirit.

However, if the cancer does not respond to treatment, or if it recurs, the consequent demoralization presents a greater challenge. In advanced disease there are three disease processes that can influence the patient's psychological response:

1. Disease may be present but dormant or growing only slowly. Some people have the capacity virtually to ignore the existence of their tumour, without denying it. They selectively attend to the non-cancer aspects of their lives. Many, however, find it frightening and frustrating to know that the cancer is still present. They cannot understand why it cannot be cut out, or why some treatment cannot be found to eradicate it. This leads to an anxious preoccupation with the current illness and its possible spread.

2. Progressive disease inevitably brings uncertainty about the effectiveness of further treatment and ultimate survival.

3. In some types of cancer treatment is effective but does not bring permanent remission. This is common in myeloma and leukaemia but may also be found with solid tumours. As recurrences mount up it becomes increasingly harder to maintain a fighting spirit.

It is not necessarily the stage of the disease as understood by the oncologist which is significant in determining a person's emotional reactions, but the stage of the disease as it is understood by the person him- or herself. Some people with advanced cancer may not have been told their prognosis or may not want to know. Their reactions will be very different from those who are fully informed e.g. knowing that metastatic breast cancer cannot be cured. But it is not only the subjective aspects of cancer at this stage that cause variation in psychological response. Different types of cancer, and even different forms of the same disease, can be associated with different prognoses. For instance, metastatic breast cancer involving the bones may be associated with much longer survival than metastatic disease in the liver or brain.

Advanced cancer can refer to people who have from 6 months to 6 years of life expectancy. Patients with advanced disease may be experiencing severe debilitating symptoms or no symptoms at all. Relatively few studies have examined the type of coping strategies used by patients with advanced disease. Classen *et al.* (1996) looked at psychological adjustment to advanced breast cancer in a sample of 101 women. As with studies of early stage cancer, fighting spirit, and emotional expressiveness were associated with better psychological adjustment. Bloom and Spiegel (1984) found avoidance coping strategies were associated with poor social functioning in women with advanced breast cancer. A few studies have made direct comparisons between the coping of patients with early and advanced disease. Greer and Watson (1987) found few differences between early and advanced stage patients in their responses to the MAC scale: both groups had similar scores for fighting spirit, helplessness, and fatalism; however, scores for anxious preoccupation were significantly higher in patients with advanced disease. Watson *et al.* (1990) found that in a small mixed cancer sample a belief in control over the course of the illness was associated with fighting spirit in early stage patients but not patients with advanced disease.

The psychological effects of physical symptoms

Despite these variations in the objective and subjective consequences of late-stage cancer, there are some factors that tend to distinguish it from early disease. One of these is the increased likelihood of physical symptoms from the cancer itself. In many of the cases we have used to illustrate therapy, the patient is living an active life with little or no apparent signs of disease. In others, physical symptoms result from the treatment they are receiving. Patients with advanced cancer may experience symptoms such as pain, breathlessness, nausea, and physical disablement. It would not

Table 12.1 Mean Mental Adjustment to Cancer (MAC) scores for patients with early- and advanced-stage disease

	Early	Advanced	
Fighting spirit	52.3	53.1	NS
Anxious preoccupations	19.5	21.7	$p < 0.001$
Fatalistic	20.8	20.0	NS
Helpless	9.4	9.6	NS
Avoidance	1.9	1.9	NS

NS = non-significant

Probability was calculated using two-tailed *t*-test.

From Greer and Watson (1987). MAC scale: Watson *et al.* (1988).

be surprising if these brought more psychological distress in their own right. Some studies (e.g. Bukberg *et al.* 1984) have demonstrated a relationship between severity of disease and psychological morbidity, but Lloyd's (1979) observation that this is not a consistent finding still holds. In a study of self-esteem in patients with breast cancer, Hodgkin's disease, and lymphoma, Greer and Burgess (1987) hypothesized that those with advanced disease would score significantly lower on self-esteem. The hypothesis was not confirmed: stage of disease was not correlated with self-esteem.

In the cognitive model it is the *interpretation* of the physical effects of the disease that causes distress. The symptoms of advanced cancer are often seen as a sign of permanent loss and a reminder to patients that they will never return to their old selves. This sense of loss may be associated with more global attributions about the self. Loss of the ability to carry out normal activities may be viewed as a sign of laziness or failure. These attributions usually imply a loss of self-worth resulting from the changes that cancer has brought. Patients feel like non-persons, as if they were being treated as dead already. This is not surprising if staff treating them, as Crary and Crary (1974) found, rate cancer worse than death. Raising the self-esteem of the patient with advanced disease can be one of the most useful contributions of APT.

Burns (1980) describes the case of a woman in her mid-40s who had disseminated lung cancer. She was weak from chemotherapy and had to give up the daily activities that had meant a great deal to her sense of identity and pride. She wrote down the following negative cognitions:

- I'm not contributing to society.
- I'm not accomplishing in my own personal realm.
- I'm not able to participate in active fun.
- I am a drain and a drag on my husband.

Burns asked her to make a graph of her personal 'worth' from the moment of birth to the moment of death (Fig. 12.1). She saw her worth as constant throughout. He then asked her to estimate her productivity over the same period. This was presented as a curve with low productivity in childhood increasing to adulthood and decreasing again later in life (Fig. 12.2). Two things then occurred to her:

First, while her illness had reduced her productivity, she still contributed to herself and her family in numerous small but nevertheless important and precious ways. Only all-or-nothing thinking could make her think her contributions were a zero.

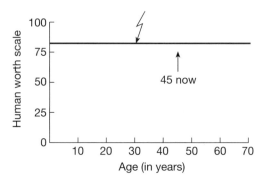

Fig. 12.1

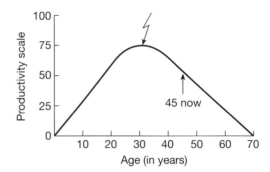

Fig. 12.2 Total contribution to society, family and self. Case report from Burns (1980).

Second, and much more important, she realized her personal worth was constant and steady: it was a given worth that was unrelated to her achievements. This meant that her human worth did not have to be earned, and she was every bit as precious in her weakened state. A smile spread across her face, and her depression melted in that moment. It was a real pleasure for me to witness and participate in this small miracle. It did not eliminate the tumour, but it did restore her missing self-esteem, and that made all the difference in the way she felt.

This brief intervention proved very effective for this woman. Burns writes: 'she died in pain but with dignity six months later'.

The concept of personal worth as a constant unchanging fact about the self may be useful for patients with advanced disease who have lost their self-esteem for similar reasons to the patient described by Burns. The next example shows how behavioural techniques can be used to combat the hopelessness which results from feeling incapacitated.

> Cathy was a 75-year-old woman who had lived with cancer of the cervix for 12 years. She had had a tremendous fighting spirit, which had helped her through several major operations. She had great faith in the surgeon who had treated her over the years. Finally the time came when further surgery was inappropriate and there was little likelihood that other treatments would work. In the past her doctors had told her what treatment she was going to have; now they asked her if she wanted to have more chemotherapy. This left her feeling anxious and abandoned. She also felt very depressed and could not stop crying. The therapist helped her to express her feelings about the change of attitude of her doctors, and tried to get her to see that her tearfulness was appropriate and normal in the circumstances. She was very clear that she wanted to get rid of her depressed mood and to get back to her old self. When the therapist investigated the cognitions associated with her mood it appeared that she was feeling ineffectual. She said that she could not lead a normal life and so felt hopeless.
>
> At the time of the interview she was being fed intravenously and was quite weak. There was only a period of a few hours when she was well enough and free to walk about. Exploring what a normal life meant to her showed a way in therapeutically. The therapist listed the things she usually enjoyed doing and then asked her which of these she could still do. The concept of all-or-nothing thinking was explained to her and the idea introduced that she could still do some, if not all, of the things that made up a normal life. She started a programme of gradually lengthening walks about the hospital, and scheduled reading and listening to the radio into her day. Her mood improved quickly following this simple intervention.

A combination of cognitive and behavioural techniques is usually required to combat this hopelessness. Cognitive techniques help to challenge the thoughts that paralyse the patient. Monitoring automatic thought may show how cognitions like: 'What's the point?' precede the decision to stay in bed instead of getting up in the morning. Weighing up the advantages and disadvantages of doing nothing often gets the patients to admit that, whether there is a point or not, they feel better if they are active. Activity scheduling and setting tasks are the behavioural homework assignments which arise from this initial cognitive intervention.

Improving quality of life

Improving the quality of life is the ultimate goal of all professionals working with patients with incurable cancer. Any palliative treatments must be measured against their toxic effects. Aggressive treatments which might be justified if there is a possibility of lengthening survival are not usually considered at this stage. Psychosocial interventions are part of the range of palliative treatments available to the oncology team. APT may have particular application in this setting because it puts so much emphasis on teaching patients to plan and organize their time so that they can maximize the quality of life.

Working with 'realistic' negative automatic thoughts

All of the methods described earlier can be used at this stage. Many of the negative thoughts experienced by the patient with advanced cancer have a realistic basis, e.g. concerning the possibility of treatment failing, the possibility of death. Although these 'realistic' negative automatic thoughts do not, at first sight, seem an appropriate focus for cognitive restructuring, there are several methods that can be used to help patients deal with them (Moorey 1996). The first step is to understand the personal meaning of the thoughts for the patient. When dealing with death, pain, and disability we all have memories and fantasies derived from our own experience of illness, which can easily get in the way of accurate understanding and empathy. Cognitive techniques can help to reduce the distorted thinking which may follow on from this. The realistic thoughts may be causing distress because they occupy a considerable amount of the person's day. Structuring the day and scheduling activities can distract the person from these ruminations. This is part of the process of helping the patient to be *life-centred* rather than *death-centred*.

There is never enough time to do all the things we want to do in life. Knowing that you have a shortened life span highlights this even further. Doing nothing is not an adaptive solution to this problem. Organizing time, making priorities and scheduling activities all contribute to the effective use of the time available and so improve quality of life. The partner should always be involved in this process, since decisions about how the couple are going to spend time together are best made jointly. Involving the partner in activity scheduling can also prevent the inadvertent undermining of homework assignments by families who try to take over more and more for the patient who is growing weaker and becoming less able.

Setting goals has another function. No one can tell patients with advanced disease how long they have to live, only that their life span is considerably shortened.

Deciding that you will be alive in 2 months' time and planning a goal to be achieved by that date is one way of dealing with this uncertainty. It can shift a future orientation which is focused solely on death into one that is focused on a life-enhancing event. Many patients spontaneously set themselves an important event in the future for which they will stay alive, e.g. a daughter's wedding, their own birthday.

Promoting fighting spirit and positive avoidance

The different adjustment styles can still apply in advanced cancer, though they may not manifest themselves in the same form. Patients with advanced cancer still show a fighting spirit. Many people rise to the challenge of treatment failure and possible death by confronting it. The patient with a fighting spirit focuses on the quality of life available and believes that he or she still has personal control. Sometimes this may extend to a determination to live as long as possible.

In advanced cancer the distinction between fighting spirit and denial may become blurred. A determination to beat cancer in the face of medical evidence that the disease is incurable could be said to demonstrate a strong fighting spirit or denial. Many patients show denial for at least some of the time during their final illness. We can summarize how the therapist can promote fighting spirit and positive avoidance in advanced disease:

- The most optimistic prognosis available from the clinician is used in promoting fighting spirit.
- The therapist helps the patient to focus on what can be achieved in life, maximizing the quality of life. Ways of presenting this might be:
  (a) 'You have tried the option of thinking about the future most of the time. What has been the result?'

      'What do you have to lose if you try spending more time on improving the quality of your life?'
  (b) 'We cannot increase the quantity of your life, but we can improve the quality'.
- The techniques described in the rest of this book are used to promote activities unrelated to cancer, but important to the patient.
- Cognitive techniques can be used to change the focus from what has been lost to what the patient still has, e.g. 'I may have cancer, but there are large bits of me which aren't affected by it. I will develop them to the utmost of my ability'.

APT as part of palliative/hospice care

Fuelled by the emergence in the late 1960s of the hospice movement, there have been many important developments in palliative medicine. Patients with end-stage cancer and other illnesses are no longer dismissed with a regretful shrug ('I am sorry but there is nothing else we can do for you'). Doctors and nurses now pay close attention to the physical and, increasingly, the emotional needs of patients who are nearing the end of their lives and continue palliative care until death. Palliative medicine has received much less publicity and far fewer resources than glamourous medical specialities, but its impact upon the quality of life of patients with incurable illness has been considerable and wholly beneficial.

The World Health Organisation (1990) has defined palliative care as 'the active total care of patients whose disease is not responsive to curative treatment, where the control of pain, of other symptoms and of psychological, social, and spiritual problems is paramount and where the goal is the best quality of life for the patient and their (sic) family'. A useful checklist of common problems in palliative care has been provided by Finlay (2000) as follows:

Physical symptoms Pain, nausea and vomiting, bowel problems and other symptoms; a common and extremely distressing symptom is breathlessness (Ahmedzai and Shrivastav 2000).

Emotional problems Depression, anxiety, fears about the future, responses to loss.

Social Financial difficulties, stress in carers, loneliness, work problems.

Spiritual issues Unanswerable questions ('Why me?', 'Is there an afterlife?'). Feelings of guilt about past events.

Family/carers What do they need to know? What will the patient allow them to be told? Can they cope with the physical and emotional demands of caring?

For many patients with end-stage disease, palliative care is provided by hospices. According to a common misconception, admission to a hospice occurs only when one is about to die. In fact, patients may be admitted on several occasions for symptom control or to provide respite for relatives who are looking after them at home. Hospices provide home care as well as treatment at the hospice, and palliative care teams to support patients and families at home or in hospital are well established throughout the UK. Studies by Hinton (1994) and Morize *et al.* (1999) have shown that during end-stage illness, anxiety and depression figure prominently among patients as well as among relatives caring for them. These symptoms can be treated in both groups by APT; but as far as psychological therapy for the patients is concerned, close collaboration with physicians and nurses in palliative care is a prerequisite, since control of physical symptoms (e.g. pain, vomiting, dyspnoea) is essential before patients can concentrate on and benefit from APT.

Terminal illness

Kausar and Akram (1998) studied 60 patients with terminal illness and 60 with non-terminal illness in India. Patients with terminal illness perceived less control over their illness, used fewer problem-focused strategies, and more emotion-focused and religion-focused coping strategies than those with non-terminal cancer.

The final stage of terminal illness begins when the patient enters a gradual decline and death is likely within weeks or months. Many of the problems encountered overlap with those seen in advanced disease and similar psychological techniques can be used. A major problem for any cognitive behavioural therapy results from the increasing limitations which the disease causes. The more limited the scope for behavioural experiments, the harder it is to construct mastery experiments. People who have had a previously good adjustment to their disease and who have had a good self-image can none the less become demoralized by the reduction in functional ability. They may respond well to cognitive techniques aimed at showing them how their worth is not dependent on their ability to function. On the other hand, patients who have had previously low self-esteem or whose self-esteem is highly dependent on external factors such as their ability to succeed in work or to help others may not respond to cognitive techniques alone. Effective cognitive therapy involves an interplay of cognitive change which is reinforced by behavioural change and in turn produces further cognitive change. Clearly, the circumstances of terminal disease limit what can be achieved by APT, but, as described below, it is still possible to alleviate the emotional distress of patients and to do so without recourse to anti-depressant drugs. It is important to remember that terminally ill patients under-report psychological distress which needs to be elicited by means of skilled sensitive clinical interviews (Lloyd-Williams and Friedman 1999).

Facing death

There is a dearth of systematic research of the experience of being close to death (Teno 1999). This is hardly surprising in view of the daunting practical problems involved in undertaking such research. Much can be learnt, however, from the comments of patients as illustrated below.

Dying man's thoughts

> Have I given enough of myself?
>
> Have I helped enough people?
>
> Have I been kind in my life?
>
> If the answer is yes,
>
> Let me die in peace.
>
> GM (1970) Personal communication

I don't want my little girl to see me like this … I want her to remember me how I looked when I was well. I hope she'll remember that I loved her. I feel so weak, I haven't the strength to bounce her up and down on my lap. I just hope Charlie and my mum will look after her properly; if I know that, I can die in peace.

B (1998) Personal communication

So, once we have recognized the limitations of the magic of doctors and medicine, where are we? We have to turn to our own magic, to our ability to 'control' our bodies … for people who have cancer, it takes the form of a conscious development of the will to live …One of the ways that all of us avoid thinking about death is by concentrating on the details of our daily lives. The work that we do every day and the people we love—the fabric of our lives—convince us that we are alive and that we will stay alive … In considering some of the talismans we all use to deny death, I don't mean to suggest that these talismans should be abandoned. However, their limits must be acknowledged … As much as I rely on my talismans—my doctors, my will, my husband, my children, and my garden peas I know that from time to time I will have to confront what Conrad has described as 'the horror'. I know that we can—all of us—confront that horror and not be destroyed by it, even to some extent be enhanced by it ... It astonishes me that having faced the terror, we continue to live, even to live with a great deal of joy ... We will never kill the dragon. But each morning we confront him. Then we give our children breakfast, perhaps put a bit more mulch on the peas, and hope that we can convince the dragon to stay away for a while longer.

Trilling (1981)

Main fears of dying patients

- Fear of the process of dying (e.g. intolerable pain).
- Fear of the consequences of death for loved ones.
- Existential fear of death itself.

Identifying the cognitive processes involved in the appraisal of death is helpful. Many patients are able to express clearly what they are afraid of, e.g. 'I can't face a painful lingering death'. Others find it more difficult. Careful questioning is needed to establish which aspects of dying are most distressing. The most valuable information can often be obtained by asking for images the patient has of death, e.g. 'I can see myself deserted by all my friends'. Exploring these ideas and the feelings associated with them can be a painful process, but it sometimes allows patients to clarify what they really fear and start anticipatory grieving.

Fear of the process of dying is by far the commonest fear and is often due to distressing past experiences of watching a relative or friend with cancer die in great pain. Fortunately, the considerable progress in pain control and in the management of other symptoms in recent years (Turner 1995) allows us to reassure these patients. However, certain symptoms of end-stage cancer such as emaciation and weakness do not respond well to currently available treatments. Fear of the consequences of death for loved ones denotes the patient's altruism. Such fears can be dealt with in cognitive therapy in joint sessions with the patient and loved one(s).

The existential fear of death itself is expressed in the question 'What will become of me after I die?' Any answer will, of course, depend on the individual's spiritual/religious beliefs. Hinton (1967) in his landmark study of dying patients reported that those with a strong religious faith and those who were non-believers were least fearful about dying; those with a faltering faith and doubts were most fearful. For patients plagued by religious doubts, referral to a minister of religion who is experienced in dealing with dying patients can be helpful. Of course, eliciting the meaning of death will depend upon the patient being willing and able to discuss death. Processes of cognitive and emotional avoidance can prevent thoughts and feelings about death from being acknowledged. Hinton (1967) describes how patients fluctuate from acceptance to denial depending on how they are feeling and to whom they are talking. Denial is not necessarily maladaptive in this respect. Hinton writes:

dying people are apt to speak or hint sombrely of the outlook at one time and talk lightly of hopeful plans soon after. Sometimes the hints that they give are fairly clear indications that they are aware of being near death ... Sometimes spontaneous disclaimers of anxiety or deliberate avoidance of reference to the future, except in the vaguest terms, show that the outcome is suspected (Hinton 1967).

The therapist must take the cue from the patient and work accordingly. Sometimes death may be an issue for discussion; at other times it will be avoided assiduously. In these situations it may be best just to listen and support.

Few of us can face death with the apparent calm of Mozart, who wrote to his father:

> Since death (properly understood) is the true ultimate purpose of our life, I have for several years past made myself acquainted with this truest and best friend of mankind so that he has for me not only nothing terrifying anymore but much that is tranquillizing and consoling! (Eissler 1955).

For most human beings, personal extinction is both frightening and unimaginable. When healthy, we live our lives without thought of death. But confronted with evidence of our mortality, we find it difficult to come to terms with the fact that, sooner or later, we will cease to exist. A contemporary British philosopher has provided a vivid description of his feelings:

> 'I was overwhelmed almost literally so, by a sense of mortality. The realization hit me like a demolition crane that I was inevitably going to die ... as in a nightmare I felt trapped and unable to escape from something that I was also unable to face. Death, my death, the literal destruction of me, was totally inevitable, and had been from the very instant of my conception ... In the face of death I craved for my life to have some meaning'. (Magee 1997)

Magee was not ill (terminally or otherwise) but was going through what he termed a mid-life crisis. The feelings he so graphically describes are rarely expressed by people who are terminally ill. As mentioned earlier, patients are far more likely to fear the process of dying and to be concerned about their loved ones. Indeed, death itself may or may not be a fearful prospect for the terminally ill. The individual's appraisal of death will depend on various factors such as his or her personal circumstances, spiritual/religious beliefs, and the degree to which adequate symptom control has been achieved. But Magee's observation regarding the need to seek meaning in one's life is of particular relevance for patients with advanced and terminal illness in their efforts to cope. Folkman (1997) has demonstrated empirically that searching for and finding positive meaning is a crucial part of the coping process. There are various ways to create positive meaning; for example making the best possible use of whatever time is left, finding that one's illness has strengthened the bond with loved ones or clarified which goals and priorities are important and which are not. For people with cancer who have young children, specific techniques for creating meaning include life-story books, letters to loved ones, audiotaped or videotaped messages, and memory boxes.

Another method of creating positive meaning is to set oneself certain goals. For patients with terminal illness, such goals may range from simple tasks which can represent an important achievement such as being able to make a cup of tea or prepare a meal for one's partner, to aiming to stay alive for long enough to see one's daughter get married. The literature contains many examples in which a strong will to live, or conversely, the loss of will to live has seemingly prolonged or reduced the length of survival well beyond that expected on clinical grounds (e.g. Selawry 1979; Maguire 1979; Greer and Watson 1987). Supporting evidence for these clinical observations comes from an epidemiological study which reported the postponement of death until symbolically meaningful occasions (Phillips and Smith 1990). Each of these ways of creating positive meaning are encouraged and form an integral part of APT.

Case example

The following case report illustrates the approach that APT takes with patients suffering from terminal illness.

> K, a 36-year-old French biochemist with testicular teratoma, was referred for psychologi-cal support. He had previously undergone an orchidectomy, chemotherapy, and surgical resection (debulking) of an abdominal mass in France. Despite this treatment, his disease was progressing, a fact of which the patient was fully aware. He had come to Britain to obtain further medical advice at The Royal Marsden Hospital.
>
> K was married with a son who was only 14 months old. The marriage was described as 'stormy' with many arguments, particularly about money. At interview, K was understand-ably depressed and anxious about his future: 'Do I have any future? I don't know'. He was also extremely angry with the doctors who, in his words, 'have put me through all this terrible treatment (chemotherapy) without any improvement in the cancer; do they really know what they are doing?' He was also angry with God for having let him get cancer as well as with his wife because she did not show enough sympathy and put their son first.
>
> The main problems identified in the initial APT session were:

- The patient's inability to decide whether to have further chemotherapy.
- Severely disturbed marital relationship.

> In order to assist the patient to make a decision regarding further chemotherapy, the therapist discussed with the oncologist details of the proposed drug regime and the likely prognosis. The oncologist recommended an aggressive chemotherapy regime which would include cisplatin; he estimated the chance of cure with this regime to be approximately 50 per cent. These details were put to the patient who was encouraged to consider carefully—in collaboration with the therapist—all the advantages and disadvantages of resuming chemotherapy. K finally decided to accept this treatment and was admitted to hospital.
>
> The second problem which had been identified, namely the disturbed marital relation-ship, was then addressed. A serious obstacle was the absence of the wife, who was living in France. She and the patient spoke on the telephone every day, and the substance of these conversations was discussed in APT sessions. No major changes could be effected; never-theless, some improvement seemed to take place after the patient agreed to put his finances in order and to make provisions for his wife and infant son.
>
> When first seen, K asked the therapist to help him develop a fighting spirit. This was done, using the techniques described in earlier chapters. In addition, the patient was given *The road back to health* to read; this book by Neil Fiore (1984) seemed particularly appropriate as the author describes his own recovery from metastatic testicular cancer. Unfortunately it soon became evident that K was not responding to chemotherapy.
>
> The goals of APT were changed. The therapist discussed with K his feelings about active treatment coming to an end and the fact that death now seemed fairly close. The therapist asked the patient what goals he regarded as important for him to accomplish before he died and how he could be helped to achieve this. He set himself the task of mak-ing financial provisions for his wife and son. Fighting spirit came to mean retaining the will to live as long as necessary to fulfil his aim. This he achieved. He was discharged from

hospital to stay with his mother who lived in London. Home care from a hospice team was provided. He was offered continuing psychological support, but declined. K died 2 weeks after discharge from hospital.

Fighting and accepting

The above case illustrates the problem of adapting fighting spirit in patients with advanced and terminal illness. The active, fighting approach of APT in the early stages of cancer must obviously be modified as the disease progresses. There comes a point where fighting to be cured or to extend life significantly becomes both unrealistic and counter-productive. Some patients are able to face this transition fairly easily. For many, however, the thought of death is so terrifying that they try to keep fighting until the very end. Handling the transition from fighting to acceptance can be a difficult task. Kath Mannix, a palliative care physician who is also a CBT therapist, suggested that one way to escape from the apparent dichotomies of fighting versus giving in and denying versus accepting, is to reframe the whole process as *fighting for*. The aim is not to fight against death, but to fight for quality of life, and this of course can go on regardless of how much time is available.

In handling this delicate phase we suggest the following guidelines:

1   The therapist should work as closely as possible with the oncologist so that both are clear about prognosis and available treatment.

2   The patient's wishes should be taken into account as much as possible. Acceptance should not be forced on a patient who is determined to fight even if the odds are against him or her.

3   The spouse/partner should be included in this final phase. The therapist must ensure that the couple are both agreed on the stance they are taking against the disease.

4   Attitudes of patient and spouse should be expected to fluctuate and not conform to a steady pattern.

Therapists who use an approach that promotes fighting spirit differ in their management of terminally ill patients. Renneker (1982) proposed helping people to fight to the end, to the extent of even getting physicians to prescribe placebo treatments. Simonton *et al.* (1978), on the other hand, placed the decision firmly in the hands of the patient. They let the patients say when they wanted to give up the fight and respect their wishes. In APT the therapist takes the patient's lead in the stance he or she wants to take. But patients who continue to fight against death often experience increasing emotional distress. For this reason, acceptance is preferable to fighting spirit at the terminal stage of cancer.

Case example

Joan was a 60-year-old social worker who had advanced cancer of the lung. She and her husband would not accept the doctor's word that there was no treatment to cure her. Her husband would say: 'Why don't they give her hope?' She desperately wanted to hear good news and would perk up if anyone said she was looking well. But this only lasted for a short time and she soon became despondent again. She was angry with God for punishing her in this way and very scared of death. None of the usual techniques of APT helped very much. Concentrating on quality of life did not work because she could not stop thinking about death. Allowing her to ventilate her feelings gave temporary relief, but in the long run only reinforced her resentment and despair. She refused to contemplate death so nothing could be done to help her face it. This woman's anxiety made the staff feel helpless. She continued to be distressed until she died.

However, such emotional distress, though common, is not inevitable in patients who fight to the end.

Case example

S, a 65-year-old man with small cell lung cancer, had undergone high dose chemotherapy with autologous bone marrow transplant. Despite this intensive treatment, which was accompanied by severe side-effects, there was no improvement in the cancer. He was told by his oncologist that no further curative treatment was available. Nevertheless, S insisted that a new experimental treatment (which he discovered on the Internet) should be tried. After discussions between the therapist, patient, and oncologist, the latter agreed to give the experimental drugs. S put up with the unpleasant physical side-effects stoically. With the encouragement of the therapist, S planned various activities that were important to him and which he was still able to carry out (e.g. writing letters). His wife consistently supported him in his wish to 'fight the cancer'. He remained emotionally calm until he developed increasing dyspnoea. He died two days later.

Working with couples

We have already emphasized the importance of including the patient's partner/spouse in APT. Although this therapy is aimed primarily at relieving emotional distress in the patient, including the partner in APT may also help the latter to cope after the patient's death. Where possible the therapist will encourage the couple to talk about death and the goals they want to achieve before they are parted. Vachon *et al.* (1977) reported that 81 per cent of widows of cancer patients who had openly discussed death before their husbands died found that talking about death made it easier to face their bereavement. After the patient's death, it is appropriate to offer the partner bereavement counselling.

The following description of APT illustrates how therapy can be applied in a terminally ill patient.

Case example

B, aged 28, was admitted to a hospice with breast cancer and liver metastases. She was referred because she had become severely depressed and refused to eat. When first seen, she would not talk to anyone. The therapist spent over an hour with her persuading her to speak. Eventually, with difficulty, she presented three main problems: (i) feeling helpless, (ii) 'I just can't eat', (iii) abdominal pain. Clearly, APT had to be integrated with palliative care, requiring close collaboration between physician, therapist, and nurses. First, adequate pain control was achieved within two days. Next, her inability to eat was tackled jointly by the therapist and nurses. In exploring this problem, it became clear that it began when eating was immediately followed by nausea. Although her nausea had gone away (due to an anti-emetic) her inability to eat persisted. She was now able to challenge the automatic thought 'I can't eat' with the response 'The sickness has gone, so perhaps

Table 12.2 Hospital and Anxiety Depression Scale (Zigmond and Smith 1983)

	Day after admission	Day after seeing her son	2 days before death
Anxiety	15	10	7
Depression	20	14	9

Scores 11–21 denote clinical anxiety and depression.

I can try to eat again'. The nurse was now able to tempt her to begin eating small amounts of food. Finally, her feelings of helplessness were addressed. B knew she did not have long to live. She felt angry that she would die so young. She felt helpless regarding her 2-year-old son: 'he won't want to see me like this … I can't do anything for him any longer'. The therapist challenged this negative automatic thought and suggested that she test it out by asking her partner to bring her son to see her. Reluctant at first, she agreed to do this. When her son saw her, he jumped on the bed and put his arms around her. She became less depressed as she realized that, despite her illness, she could still be a mother to her son for brief periods.

Because she felt increasingly weak, therapy sessions had to be geared to her physical state and be fairly brief (30 minutes maximum). Nevertheless, her psychological response was obvious (see Table 12.2). One main fear remained, namely, what would happen to her son when she died? Her partner was not the biological father and had not legally adopted him. The therapist held a joint session with B and her partner; they agreed to legal adoption and the next day, a solicitor arranged this. She was encouraged to make an audiotape for her son. B died five days later.

Organic causes of psychological disturbance

Before we end this chapter, we must sound a note of caution. Psychological disturbance can arise from the physiological effects of cancer itself or from the side-effects of opioids and certain chemotherapeutic drugs (see Chapter 1). Delirium (acute confusional state) is common in patients with advanced and, especially, terminal cancer. This disorder which is often mistaken for anxiety or depression (Levine *et al.* 1978; Breitbart and Cohen 1998), requires urgent medical treatment (Greer 1995). Therefore, the therapist who is not medically qualified is advised to proceed with caution when commencing APT with patients suffering from advanced or terminal cancer. It is important to consider the possibility of an organic cause for the patient's psychological symptoms and to request a specialist neuropsychiatric opinion if there is any doubt.

Summary

As an integral component of palliative care, cognitive behaviour therapy can be used to improve the quality of life of patients with advanced and terminal cancer. As the disease progresses, it becomes more difficult to conduct formal APT because of patients' increasing infirmity. Nevertheless, it is still possible to reduce emotional distress by the cognitive and behavioural methods described in this chapter.

Chapter 13

Group therapy

Individual versus group therapy

David Spiegel, a pioneer of group therapy for cancer patients, has put forward three advantages of group therapy (Spiegel *et al.* 1999):

- social (i.e. emotional) support which patients give each other;
- 'helper–therapy principle'—i.e. patients gain self-esteem through their ability to help others in the group;
- cost effectiveness.

The last-mentioned advantage is, of course, self-evident. But, despite increasing pressure (both in the UK and the US) from those who hold the purse strings and who know the cost of everything but the value of nothing, money should not be the deciding factor. We would agree that the first two advantages listed by Spiegel are undoubtedly important considerations in favour of group therapy. On the other hand, therapy with individual patients together with their partners (APT)—as described by us— also has certain advantages. First, it is widely recognized that the effects of cancer involve not only the patient but also his or her loved ones (e.g. Baider *et al.* 1996) and that it is important to involve the latter in the patient's cancer care (Speice *et al.* 2000); this is achieved with APT. Second, an inconvenient fact not mentioned in the literature on group therapy is that by no means all patients wish to join a group; some prefer individual psychotherapy. Indeed, there are often considerable difficulties in recruiting cancer patients to group therapy; refusal rates as high as 69 per cent (Ford *et al.* 1990) and even 80 per cent (Edelman *et al.* 1999b) have been reported. The answer is clear: both individual and group therapy should be made available and patients should be given a choice.

In Chapter 3, our review of clinical trials revealed that psychological therapy can improve the quality of life (psychosocial adjustment) of patients with cancer significantly and such improvement has been documented in trials of both group and individual therapy including APT. Only two investigations, to date, have directly compared group with individual counselling. Cain and her colleagues (1986) randomly assigned a consecutive series of women with gynaecological cancers to routine care, individual counselling, and group counselling respectively. Counselling consisted of eight sessions during which patients discussed their fears, were informed about their cancers and advised about diet, physical exercise, and sexual functioning; they were also given relaxation training, encouraged to express their feelings to caregivers and family and to develop short and long-term goals. Six months after counselling, patients in both counselling groups had significantly improved psychosocial adjustment compared to controls. Individual and group counselling were found to be equally beneficial.

Fawzy *et al.* (1996) allocated 104 patients with newly diagnosed malignant melanoma to either six sessions of group cognitive behaviour therapy, six sessions of individual cognitive behaviour therapy, or assessment only. Again the group and individual treatments were equally effective and superior to the control condition. At 1 year follow-up the group treatment actually produced more improvement than individual therapy on a measure of coping skills.

In a meta-analysis of trials which sought to alleviate anxiety and/or depression in people with cancer, Sheard and Maguire (1999) found group and individual therapy to be equally effective (see Chapter 3).

Models of group therapy

Various kinds of group therapy run by professionals for cancer patients have been described.

Psychoeducational groups concentrate on teaching patients about their cancers and the treatments they are receiving. In addition coping skills, stress management, and relaxation exercises are often taught. Therapy is brief, usually about six to eight weeks. Examples of psychoeducational group therapy programmes which have been evaluated in randomized trials include studies by Weisman *et al.* (1980), Johnson (1982), Cain *et al.* (1986; see above), Cunningham and Tocco (1989), Fawzy *et al.* (1990a), and Berglund *et al.* (1994).

Supportive-expressive group therapy has been developed by Spiegel and his colleagues (1981, 1989) and details of the techniques used have been published in the form of a manual (Spiegel and Spira 1991). In summary, groups of 7–10 women with metastatic breast cancer met weekly for a year. During these meetings, patients discussed: their cancer treatments, family and communication problems, learning to live with terminal illness, and issues of dying and death. Emphasis was placed on expressing feelings and fears about their disease and on mutual support and learning from each other, the so-called 'helper–therapy principle'.

Cognitive-behavioural methods have been adapted to meet the specific needs of patients with cancer in the form of individual therapy (Moorey and Greer 1989) and subsequently in the form of group therapy (Kissane *et al.* 1997; Edelman *et al.* 1999b). The characteristics of individual therapy (APT) described in detail earlier—namely focusing on specific current problems, identifying and challenging negative automatic thoughts, setting goals, developing coping skills, scheduling of activities that provide a sense of achievement and of pleasure, relaxation training and encouraging expression of emotions—can be applied in group therapy.

The three broad categories of group therapy described here are neither sharply defined nor mutually exclusive. In practice, clinicians sometimes combine elements from more than one type of therapy. For example, Cunningham and Tocco's (1989)

Table 13.1 Group cognitive behavioural interventions in cancer

Education about cancer[1,4]

Relaxation[1,2,3,4,5]

Positive mental imagery[3]

Goal setting[3,5]

Physical activity[1]

Pleasant events scheduling[2]

Lifestyle management[3]

Problem solving[2,4]

Communication and assertion[2,5]

Feelings management[2]

Stress management[2]

Coping skills training[4]

Monitoring and challenging negative automatic thoughts[2,3,5]

Psychological support[2,4]

[1]Heinrich and Schag 1985; [2]Telch and Telch 1986; [3]Cunningham and Tocco 1989, Edmonds *et al.* 1999; [4]Fawzy *et al.* 1990a, 1993; [5]Edelman *et al.* 1999b.

group therapy combined psychoeducational methods with supportive discussions and some cognitive-behavioural methods. One apparent difference between the various types of group therapy is the duration of treatment: psychoeducational and cognitive-behavioural therapies are usually brief interventions (about 6–12 sessions) whereas in Spiegel's supportive-expressive groups, therapy was continued for a whole year. That study, however, involved women with advanced disease (Spiegel *et al.* 1989); recently, Spiegel *et al.* (1999) have conducted supportive-expressive group therapy for women with recently diagnosed breast cancer for 12 weekly sessions only.

Table 13.1 summarizes the techniques that have been used in seven of the outcome studies of group cognitive behaviour therapy for people with cancer. The most common interventions have been relaxation, monitoring and challenging automatic thoughts, education about cancer, goal setting, problem solving, communication and assertion, stress management, and psychological support.

What group therapies have in common

Most of these different models of group therapy share certain important characteristics:

♦ Mutual support which patients give each other is the bedrock of all types of group therapy; one practical consequence of this is that, in contrast to group therapy in psychiatric practice, cancer patients are encouraged to maintain contact with each other outside the group sessions.

♦ The therapist focuses with the group on current problems.

♦ The therapist facilitates interaction between members of the group.

- Open expression of feelings is encouraged.
- Through the group process, the therapist fosters the development of active coping strategies. This usually begins (as in individual therapy) with information and emotion-focused coping followed by problem-focused resolution of patients' current concerns (Spiegel *et al.* 1999), and finally encouraging meaning-based coping to promote psychological well-being (Folkman and Greer 2000).

Therapy for all or selected patients?

Should all patients who develop cancer or only those showing evidence of emotional distress receive psychological therapy? A common sense approach should be adopted towards this perennial question. In our clinical experience (in the UK), cancer patients who show only minor or no evidence of psychological morbidity are, understandably, likely to decline invitations to take part in psychotherapy. The needs of these patients are best served by trained oncology counsellors—usually nurses—who will provide information or explanations as requested. By contrast, patients who need, and are likely to benefit from, psychological therapy are those who experience persistent emotional distress, who feel helpless and hopeless, and who are clinically anxious or depressed. Indeed the studies that have treated these high risk groups seem to achieve better results (Sheard and Maguire 1999). Such patients can be identified by means of psychological screening instruments such as those developed by Weisman *et al.* (1980), Greer and Watson (1987), Zabora *et al.* (1990), and Watson *et al.* (1994).

Practical considerations

Having decided to set up a group therapy service, a number of practical issues need to be considered. How many patients should be included in the group? Should the group be open (i.e. new patients can join at any time) or closed (i.e. once the group is formed and for the duration of therapy no new patients can join)? Should patients with different cancers at various stages of disease be included or should any given group be confined to patients with the same type of cancer and disease stage? At which stages during the course of cancer should therapy be offered? Lastly, how long should therapy be continued? To these questions, no definitive, evidence-based answers can be given. There are, however, several detailed informative descriptions of group therapy in the literature (e.g. Spiegel and Spira 1991; Kissane *et al.* 1997; Spira 1998; Edelman *et al.* 1999b; Feigin *et al.* 2000) that provide useful guidelines.

Therapy is usually conducted with 6–12 patients in closed or semi-closed groups. In both cases, patients commit themselves to an agreed number of sessions. Closed groups are more suitable for short-term therapy, but where long-term therapy is planned—particularly with patients who suffer from advanced disease—the likelihood of a high drop-out rate due to increasing infirmity or death precludes a closed group. Under these circumstances, a semi-closed group to which new patients can be invited in place of those who leave is the best option. With regard to diagnosis and stage of disease, nearly all therapists (Weisman *et al.* 1980 are an exception) favour groups comprising patients with the same cancer at a similar stage of disease. The advantages of homogeneous groups, whose members have much in common, are obvious. But when it comes to uncommon cancers, it may not be possible to find sufficient numbers of patients to form such groups (Spira 1998). To overcome this practical problem Spira advocates mixed groups consisting of patients with a variety of cancers at various stages of disease. Mixed groups, however, present considerable difficulties because these individuals often have widely differing needs. A better solution, in our view, is individual therapy for these patients.

Lastly, we turn to the timing and duration of therapy. Although both these factors may well affect the outcome of therapy, neither has been subjected to controlled clinical trials. Clinical experience suggests that the occasions when therapy is most commonly needed are: (i) immediately after initial diagnosis, (ii) at recurrence or evidence of advancing disease, and (iii) during terminal illness. However, since individual patients will require psychological intervention at varying times depending on their particular circumstances, psychotherapy should be made available at every stage of the cancer process (Sellick and Crooks 1999). As far as duration of therapy is concerned, there are wide variations from weekly sessions for 4 weeks (Weisman *et al.* 1980) up to a whole year (Spiegel *et al.* 1981). The optimum number of sessions has not been determined empirically, but it is obvious that this will vary according to the individual needs of patients and the stage of the disease. Generally speaking, brief therapy is appropriate for patients with early cancer whereas patients with more advanced disease will require more prolonged therapy.

Comparing group therapies

We have previously described studies of the effect of psychological therapy (individual and group) on quality of life and on survival. The question arises as to which model of group therapy provides the best results. As far as survival is concerned, no studies comparing different kinds of group therapy have been reported. With regard to quality of life, a comprehensive meta-analytical study of psychological interventions (individual and group combined) revealed that such interventions significantly improved emotional adjustment, functional adjustment as well as disease—and treatment-related symptoms, but there were no significant differences in outcome between various kinds of intervention (Meyer and Mark 1995). The authors point out, however, that their results were based on studies comparing psychological treatment with no treatment controls; they recommend studies which compare different therapies directly.

Very few such studies have been published. Cunningham and Tocco (1989) compared psychoeducational group therapy including training in coping skills with supportive therapy which included supportive discussions, ventilation of feelings, and information sharing. The patients had various cancers, the commonest being breast cancer. Greater improvement in affective symptoms occurred in the group that received coping skills training than among patients who received supportive intervention only. Similar results were reported by Telch and Telch (1986) who compared group coping skills training with supportive group therapy and a no-therapy group in patients with various cancers who showed 'marked psychosocial distress'. Results demonstrated a consistent superiority of the coping skills intervention over supportive group therapy and the no-treatment control. Bottomley *et al.* (1996), in a small pilot study assigned newly diagnosed, psychologically distressed cancer patients to either a cognitive-behavioural group, a social support group, or a non-intervention group. Results showed that cognitive-behavioural therapy was superior to social support in improving patients' coping styles. These few studies provide some preliminary evidence suggesting that cognitive-behavioural methods may be more successful than supportive discussions in group therapy. Such evidence, however, is insufficient to permit firm conclusions to be drawn.

An interesting suggestion has been put forward by Bloch and Kissane (1995). They argue that cognitive-behaviour therapy may be more applicable to early stage disease to help patients to adjust to their potential 'survivorship'. Supportive-expressive therapy, on the other hand, encourages sharing of feelings about existential concerns and may, for that reason, be more suited to patients with metastatic disease. Bloch and Kissane's suggestion requires empirical testing. A different approach has been recommended by a leading researcher and therapist who has personally experienced and survived cancer:

> 'It surely makes sense to use therapies combining all the modalities that responsible therapists have described as helping patients. There is no room for partisanship here' (Cunningham 1999).

In the light of the inadequate current state of knowledge, Cunningham's recommendation seems reasonable. But this is not a satisfactory state of affairs. We need to know which specific psychotherapeutic procedures produce measurable improvement in psychosocial adjustment and which patients are most—and least—likely to benefit from the various components of group therapy.

Summary and conclusions

1 Both individual and group psychotherapy should be made available for cancer patients who, on psychological screening, show evidence of persistent emotional distress (clinical anxiety, depression, helplessness/hopelessness).

2 Group therapy conducted with cancer patients can be categorized under three headings: psychoeducational, supportive-expressive, and cognitive-behavioural. There is some overlap between these models.

3 Studies comparing the models of group therapy are rare. Preliminary evidence suggests an advantage for cognitive-behavioural therapy, but further studies are required before any firm conclusions can be drawn.

4 Homogeneous groups (i.e. patients with the same cancer and stage of disease) consisting of 6–12 members are recommended.

5 Therapy is required most commonly following the diagnosis of cancer, at recurrence, and during terminal illness, but therapy should be available throughout the course of cancer.

6   The duration of therapy in the literature varies widely. Clinical experience suggests that patients with early cancer can benefit from brief therapy whereas more prolonged therapy is required for patients with advanced or terminal illness.

Studies are required to determine: (a) the comparative effectiveness of different models of group therapy and (b) the optimum times and duration for psychological intervention.

Chapter 14

Concluding remarks

In this book we have tried to achieve a balance between theory, research data, and practical comment, updating the original edition in each area. The prevailing emphasis remains, none the less, on the clinical applications of cognitive behavioural techniques to people with cancer. Despite the large quantity of work demonstrating the effectiveness of CBT for people with cancer, there are still relatively few practical texts describing 'how to do it'. Inevitably we have not been able to cover the whole area of psychosocial oncology. We have not tried to review all the studies of psychological morbidity in cancer, nor have we attempted to draw together the increasing body of data concerning coping. Instead we have, in the first chapter, used some of the research evidence to illustrate the model of adjustment to cancer which forms the basis of adjuvant psychological therapy (APT). Chapters 3 and 4 contain comprehensive current reviews of the literature concerning the efficacy of cognitive behavioural interventions in cancer and the evidence that mental adjustment may influence disease outcome. The second half of the book has used the model described in the first part as the framework for a practical guide to psychotherapy for patients with cancer.

Although the effectiveness of adjuvant psychological therapy has been demonstrated further questions need to be answered. These include questions about what are the effective components of the treatment package, whether, as the evidence suggests, APT is more effective than other forms of therapy such as counselling, and which patients are most likely to benefit. Perhaps most importantly, we need to find a way to disseminate the techniques that have been shown to be effective in randomized controlled trials carried out by experts to clinical situations. There is some preliminary evidence that cognitive therapy can be learned by palliative care nurses with no previous psychotherapy training. Developing brief training packages so that oncology professionals can apply some of the components of APT in their everyday practice is probably the most important contribution cognitive behaviour therapy can make to psycho-oncology.

Appendix I

Coping with Cancer

Everyone learns to deal with cancer in their own individual way, bringing their unique strengths and resources to the process of coping. There are as many different reactions to cancer as there are people with the illness. Psychological therapy is about helping you to find what works best for you. This may mean exploring new ways to think about the disease and its impact on your life, trying new methods to cope with the illness, or even just getting back to some of the things you used to do before the cancer came along. How people cope seems to depend very much on how they view themselves and their illness. Disturbing thoughts and feelings, such as anger, guilt and fear, are common: they are part of the process of coming to terms with cancer. Here are some examples of the sorts of thoughts and emotions that you might have had:

Thoughts	Emotion
Why me? I've done nothing to deserve this.	Anger
Why do I feel so tired? Has the cancer really gone?	Fear
Will people avoid me because I've got the big C?	Fear and shame
There's nothing I can do. It's hopeless.	Depression
I'm not a normal person any more.	Depression
I know that I can deal with this, with the help of my family and the doctors.	Hope

Some reactions, like the last one, can help you live life to the full and fight back against the cancer. Others, if they persist, can make it harder to cope. You probably have a mixture of the two sorts. You may think that reactions like this are 'just part of you' and cannot be changed, but, as the rest of this leaflet explains, by working on how you think and what you do it is possible to have a stronger and more comfortable way of coping.

Psychological therapy

The psychological therapy which you are starting can help you to cope better, in partnership with any physical treatments you may be having. It takes about 6 to 12 hourly sessions once a week. Your therapist will help you to identify the problems you face and your strengths and weaknesses in dealing with them. You can then decide together which problems to tackle and how best to do this. If you have a partner, you may choose for him or her to come to some of the sessions: some of the problems you have may best be overcome by the two of you working together.

Some of the methods used are set out below. Some will be helpful to you, others may not. You and your therapist will decide which to try, and you will learn how and when to use them. As you read about them, think about whether they could be useful to you. With what sort of problems might they be helpful?

Problem solving

You are probably already a very good problem-solver, but cancer can make you feel paralysed. Once you have identified the problems you want to work on, you can think of possible solutions with the help of your therapist. Your partner can make a contribution to your coping, and you will have another set of ideas on what to do. You will learn to decide which solution to try first, and then be helped to put it into practice.

For instance, many people feel tongue-tied when seeing their doctor and forget all the important questions they want to ask. Other patients who have used the therapy have come up with a number of solutions using problem solving with their therapist or partner:

1 Write down what you want to ask, and read it out.
2 Bring someone with you to the consultation.
3 Rehearse what you want to say with your therapist or partner.

You can probably think of more. Therapy is about enabling you to recover your confidence to be an effective problem-solver.

Expressing feelings

You may well have strong, unpleasant feelings such as fear, sadness, or anger. You may not want to burden other people with them or feel unsafe to express them but research suggests that being open about how you feel can help you to cope better. You will have the chance to talk about such feelings with your therapist and to improve communication with important people in your life so that you can support each other better.

Dealing with negative thoughts

When coping with cancer, you may face very unpleasant experiences, major changes in your way of life and uncertainty about the future. When you think about these things, some of your thoughts will help you cope, whereas others may be unhelpful and lead to distress. Once you have faced your negative emotions and shared them with your therapist, you can start to explore the thoughts behind them. Some examples of thoughts which make it more difficult to cope are:

'I know I'm going to die from the cancer'.
'There's no point in doing anything'.
'No one will love me if my hair falls out'.
'I can't cope'.

Such thoughts can lead you to underestimate your coping abilities and overestimate your problems; we call them negative automatic thoughts because they are unrealistically pessimistic and because they seem to come from nowhere and 'automatically' pop into your mind. In therapy you will learn to separate realistic negative thoughts from extreme or unhelpful negative thoughts. They are difficult to spot to start with (you are probably not aware that you have them) and the first step is to learn to recognize them. You can keep a diary of when you get these thoughts, what might have triggered them and what you feel and do when they come into your mind. Many people find that just catching the thoughts allows them to get more control over them, but if you are feeling very anxious or depressed this may not work in itself. You may need more help from the therapist to change the patterns of self-defeating thinking. You can start to ask yourself questions to examine how realistic or helpful these negative thoughts really are, and start to find alternative, more constructive ways to think. Research has shown that doing this can improve your mood and make you feel more in control of your situation. Here is an example of how this works:

> A man with cancer felt a twinge in his hip. He immediately thought: 'I've got cancer in my bones'. This is a negative automatic thought—he had jumped to the worst possible conclusion. Not surprisingly, he felt anxious. He questioned his reason for believing this and remembered that he had had this pain on and off for years—long before he got cancer. He was able to challenge the thought with the reply: 'I had arthritis in my hip long before I got cancer. The last check-up showed the cancer hadn't spread. These are just ordinary aches and pains'. This reduced the belief that the cancer had spread and so he felt less anxious.

Do not worry if this seems complicated. If you and your therapist decide to use this technique, you will learn it gradually, using examples from your own negative thoughts.

Improving the quality of life

The goal of all our therapy is to improve the quality of your life. When you have cancer, you may miss out on some of things you enjoy. This may be because of physical ill-health, because you spend a lot of time thinking about your illness and its treatment or because you do not see the point in going on with ordinary life. You can reduce the effect the illness has on you and fight back by doing things you enjoy and things which give you a sense of achievement. We have found that this gives people back a feeling of being in control of their lives. It also makes them feel connected with the real world, so they are a person in their own right and not just a 'cancer patient.' Your therapist may help you to keep a diary of what you are doing that is pleasurable or that gives you a feeling of achievement. You can build on this by planning challenging and enjoyable activities into your week. It is important to set your expectations at the right level—if you are tired and weak, making a cup of tea may be a major achievement in itself. If you are unable to do everything as before, do not give up: do what you can and above all give yourself credit for it. You and your therapist will discuss ways to use your time and energy to best advantage.

Learning new coping methods

There are several other coping methods as well as the ones we have already mentioned. Depending on your problems, your therapist may suggest other techniques. Many people find practising relaxation helpful. Physical tension and distress can build up in a vicious circle where each increases the other. You and your therapist may decide to try to break the circle with relaxation exercises. You will learn them either from a tape or from your therapist and practise them regularly. Being able to relax may help you to deal with stressful situations.

Conclusions

You may be coping very well already, but have a few problems or worries, or you may be in great difficulties and doubt that you will ever overcome them. Whatever your situation, you and your therapist can work together alongside your other treatments to help you to cope with cancer and to ensure that you are still in control of your life.

You may find it helpful to read this leaflet again now, picking up the points that you think apply to you and any with which you disagree. Your therapist will be happy to talk about any questions or concerns you may have about this therapy and how you can use it.

Tick a box if you think one of these could be helpful to you:

Problem solving ☐

Expressing feelings ☐

Dealing with negative thoughts ☐

Improving the quality of life ☐

Learning new coping methods ☐

Would you be willing to practise self-help assignments between sessions?

I am willing to practise self-help
   assignments between sessions ☐

Appendix II

Thinking errors

When people feel overwhelmed or demoralized they often get things out of proportion. This can lead them to exaggerate the real problems they are facing, and to underestimate their ability to cope with these problems. In these situations a person's thinking shows certain 'negative distortions', or 'thinking errors'. Some of the examples below may help you to recognize the distortions in your negative thoughts.

1. Overgeneralization

This distortion means that you see a single negative event as a never-ending pattern of defeat. For instance, if you have a row with your partner the day after you get back from hospital you think: 'It's the cancer. We'll always be arguing, things will never be the same again. We might as well split up now and get it over with'.

2. Magnification and minimization

You exaggerate the importance of some things, such as other patient's strengths and coping abilities, while at the same time playing down others until they appear insignificant, such as your own methods of coping. You may say to yourself: 'Everyone is coping better than me. I'm just a heap'.

3. All-or-nothing thinking

The world is seen in absolute, black and white terms. If your performance falls short of perfect you see yourself as a complete failure, or if the treatment is not 100% likely to be successful you see it as useless.

For example, a man who had been told that he could not be cured of cancer said: 'If I can't be cured, there's no point in doing anything. I might as well die now'. With appropriate treatment he could have months or years of active life.

4. Selective attention

If you feel depressed you are only able to think about the negative parts of your life. You selectively attend to these while ignoring all the positive things that are happening to you.

For example, a woman with breast cancer who was about to receive chemotherapy could only think of the side-effects that she would experience over the course of treatment. She thought of the unpleasantness of the next few months and ignored the fact that if the treatment was successful she would be able to enjoy the rest of her life. By focusing on this she also failed to see what she was able to do and to enjoy on a day-to-day basis.

5. Negative predictions

The future for many people with cancer is uncertain. But you can turn this into a negative certainty by assuming the worst:

'I know this treatment won't work.'

'I won't be able to cope if the cancer comes back.'

'If I lose my hair as a result of this treatment, my partner will no longer find me attractive.'

'Even if I'm cured of cancer I know something else will come along to cause problems for me.'

6. Mind-reading

Instead of finding out what people are thinking you jump to conclusions; but attempts to read other people's minds are rarely successful.

For example, a patient who had been successfully treated for cancer of the salivary gland felt herself to be under great stress at home. She thought that her family were deliberately not helping her because they were lazy and didn't care about her. In fact, they had wrongly assumed that once she was physically well everything could get back to normal immediately; they were acting out of ignorance, not malice.

7. Shoulds and oughts

You try to motivate yourself with 'shoulds' and 'oughts', but end up feeling guilty. For example, 'I should be able to do everything I did before I got cancer. Even though I don't feel well, I should still be looking after my children.'

When you direct 'should' statements towards others or life in general you feel anger and resentment: 'My husband and daughter should know I'm under stress and treat me differently'.

'I have tried to live a good life, I shouldn't have got cancer'.

8. Labelling

You apply a critical label to yourself instead of accurately describing the situation. Instead of saying: 'I didn't do that job as well as I might have done' you say to yourself: 'I'm a failure'. Or if you find it difficult to concentrate because of the stress you are under you say: 'I'm an idiot'.

9. Personalization

You see yourself as the cause of some negative event for which you are not necessarily responsible. If your children are badly behaved you say to yourself: 'It must be my fault'. If friends cancel a visit you say: 'It must be because I have cancer'.

Identifying negative thoughts is the first step in learning to change your thinking. Real negative events can be exaggerated and distorted until they seem enormous problems which you cannot hope to solve. If you master the thinking errors you can cut your problems down to size, and devote your energy to solving them rather than just worrying about them.

Appendix III

Weekly Activity Schedule

Time	Monday	Tuesday	Wednesday	Thursday	Friday	Saturday	Sunday
9–10							
10–11							
11–12							
12–1							
1–2							
2–3							
3–4							
4–5							
5–6							
6–7							
7–8							
8–12							

Appendix IV

Thought Record

Situation	Physical sensations (rate from 0–10)	Emotions (rate from 0–10)	Automatic thoughts	Alternative response	Action plan

Appendix Va

Mental Adjustment to Cancer (MAC) Scale

Name:

Date: _____

A number of statements are given below which describe people's reactions to having cancer. Please circle the appropriate number to the right of each statement, indicating how far it applies to you at present. For example, if the statement definitely does *not* apply to you then you should circle 1 in the first column.

	Definitely does not apply to me	Does *not* apply to me	Applies to me	Definitely applies to me
1. I have been doing things that I believe will improve my health, e.g. I have changed my diet	1	2	3	4
2. I feel I can't do anything to cheer myself up	1	2	3	4
3. I feel that problems with my health prevent me from planning ahead	1	2	3	4
4. I believe that my positive attitude will benefit my health	1	2	3	4
5. I don't dwell on my illness	1	2	3	4
6. I firmly believe that I will get better	1	2	3	4
7. I feel that nothing I can do will make any difference	1	2	3	4
8. I've left it all to my doctors	1	2	3	4

9. I feel that life is hopeless	1	2	3	4
10. I have been doing things that I believe will improve my health, e.g. exercised	1	2	3	4
11. Since my cancer diagnosis I now realize how precious life is and I'm making the most of it	1	2	3	4
12. I've put myself in the hands of God	1	2	3	4
13. I have plans for the future, e.g. holiday, jobs, housing	1	2	3	4
14. I worry about the cancer returning or getting worse	1	2	3	4
15. I've had a good life; what's left is a bonus	1	2	3	4
16. I think my state of mind can make a lot of difference to my health	1	2	3	4
17. I feel that there is nothing I can to help myself	1	2	3	4
18. I try to carry on my life as I've always done	1	2	3	3
19. I would like to make contact with others in the same boat	1	2	3	
20. I am determined to put it all behind me	1	2	3	4
21. I have difficulty in believing that this has happened to me	1	2	3	4
22. I suffer a great anxiety about it	1	2	3	4
23. I am not very hopeful about the future	1	2	3	4
24. At the moment I take one day at a time	1	2	3	4

(continued)

	Definitely does *not* apply to me	Does *not* apply to me	Applies to me	Definitely applies to me
25. I feel like giving up	1	2	3	4
26. I try to keep a sense of humour about it	1	2	3	4
27. Other people worry about me more than I do	1	2	3	4
28. I think of other people who are worse off	1	2	3	4
29. I am trying to get as much information as I can about cancer	1	2	3	4
30. I feel that I can't control what is happening	1	2	3	4
31. I try to have a very positive attitude	1	2	3	4
32. I keep quite busy, so I don't have time to think about it	1	2	3	4
33. I avoid finding out more about it	1	2	3	4
34. I see my illness as a challenge	1	2	3	4
35. I feel fatalistic about it	1	2	3	4
36. I feel completely at a loss about what to do	1	2	3	4
37. I feel very angry about what has happened to me	1	2	3	4
38. I don't really believe I have cancer	1	2	3	4
39. I count my blessings	1	2	3	4
40. I try to fight the illness	1	2	3	4

(Watson and Greer 1988)

Courtauld Emotional Control (CEC) Scale

Entry date: _____

Patient name: Mrs/Ms/Mr _____ Age: _____

Occupation: _____

Listed below are some of the reactions people have to certain feelings or emotions. Read through the items on each list and, by circling an appropriate number on the scale indicate how far each describes the way you *generally* react.

For example: In reaction A, if you think you *almost never* keep quiet when you feel angry or annoyed, then you would circle 1.

Please circle a number for every reaction from A through to U. Work quickly and circle only one number on each line.

When I feel angry (very annoyed)	Almost never	Sometimes	Often	Almost always
A. I keep quiet	1	2	3`	4
B. I refuse to argue or say anything	1	2	3	4
C. I bottle it up	1	2	3	4
D. I say what I feel	1	2	3	4
E. I avoid making a scene	1	2	3	4
F. I smother my feelings	1	2	3	4
G. I hide my annoyance	1	2	3	4

When I feel anxious (worried)	Almost never	Sometimes	Often	Almost always
H. I let others see how I feel	1	2	3	4
I. I keep quiet	1	2	3	4
J. I refuse to say anything about it	1	2	3	4
K. I tell others about it	1	2	3	4
L. I say what I feel	1	2	3	4
M. I bottle it up	1	2	3	4
N. I smother my feelings	1	2	3	4

When I feel unhappy (miserable)	Almost never	Sometimes	Often	Almost always
O. I refuse to say anything about it	1	2	3	4
P. I hide my unhappiness	1	2	3	4
Q. I put on a bold face	1	2	3	4
R. I keep quiet	1	2	3	4
S. I let others see how I feel	1	2	3	4
T. I smother my feelings	1	2	3	4
U. I bottle it up	1	2	3	4

(Watson and Greer 1983)

Please check that you have circled *one* number on each line and that you have circled a number for *every* reaction, from A through to U.

Thank you

Cancer Coping Questionnaire (21-item version)

Name................................   Hospital number...................

People have many ways of coping with the stress that cancer puts them under. How stressful has the last week been for you?

Very stressful   Moderately stressful   Slightly stressful   Not at all stressful

☐   ☐   ☐   ☐

Have you worried about cancer in the last week?

Most of the time   A lot of the time   Some of the time   None of the time

☐   ☐   ☐   ☐

On the following pages there is a list of different methods for coping. Think about how you have coped with your illness in the *last week* and circle how often you have used each method described. No one uses all the ways of coping described, but everyone uses some of them.

IN THE LAST WEEK DID YOU:

	Very often	Often	Sometimes	Not at all
1. Make definite plans for the future?	4	3	2	1
2. Try breathing slowly and deeply to cope with anxiety?	4	3	2	1
3. Distract yourself from worrying thoughts?	4	3	2	1
4. Remind yourself that aches and pains could be caused by things other than the cancer spreading?	4	3	2	1
5. Make a list of priorities for the week so that you got important things done?	4	3	2	1
6. Stand back to get the seriousness of your illness into proportion?	4	3	2	1

	Very often	Often	Sometimes	Not at all
7. Look for what strengths you have to cope with cancer?	4	3	2	1
8. Cope with frustration by channeling it into other things (e.g. physical activity like housework or gardening)?	4	3	2	1
9. Remind yourself of what things you still have in life despite of cancer?	4	3	2	1
10. Organize your day so that you got the most out of it, despite of cancer?	4	3	2	1
11. Practise relaxation?	4	3	2	1
12. Answer back worrying thoughts?	4	3	2	1
13. Plan your day so that you got on with some activities unrelated to cancer?	4	3	2	1
14. Make sure you thought of some of the positive aspects of your life?	4	3	2	1

If you are in a close relationship, think of how you and your partner have coped in the last week.

IN THE LAST WEEK DID YOU:

	Very often	Often	Sometimes	Not at all
15. Involve your partner in an activity that helped you cope with cancer?	4	3	2	1
16. Talk with your partner about the impact of cancer on your lives?	4	3	2	1
17. Ask your partner what (s)he was thinking, rather than making assumptions?	4	3	2	1
18. Try to see cancer as a challenge that you and your partner have to face together?	4	3	2	1
19. Discuss how your partner could help support you?	4	3	2	1
20. Talk to your partner about how you could organize things to take some pressure off you (e.g. changing who does household chores)?	4	3	2	1
21. Think of how cancer had brought you and your partner closer together?	4	3	2	1

Cancer Concerns Checklist

Copyright © CRC

We would like to know the different concerns that may have been worrying you about your illness and treatment over the last few weeks. Please remember to answer all the questions.

Tick only one box in each section

The illness itself (what is it, is it better etc)

- [ ] Not a worry
- [ ] Slightly worried
- [ ] Moderately worried
- [ ] Very worried
- [ ] Extremely worried

Feeling different from other people

- [ ] Not a worry
- [ ] Slightly worried
- [ ] Moderately worried
- [ ] Very worried
- [ ] Extremely worried

Treatment for the illness

- [ ] Not a worry
- [ ] Slightly worried
- [ ] Moderately worried
- [ ] Very worried
- [ ] Extremely worried

How I feel about myself as a man or woman

- [ ] Not a worry
- [ ] Slightly worried
- [ ] Moderately worried
- [ ] Very worried
- [ ] Extremely worried

How I have been feeling physically

- [ ] Not a worry
- [ ] Slightly worried
- [ ] Moderately worried
- [ ] Very worried
- [ ] Extremely worried

My relationship with my partner

- [ ] Not a worry
- [ ] Slightly worried
- [ ] Moderately worried
- [ ] Very worried
- [ ] Extremely worried

Not being able to do things

- [ ] Not a worry
- [ ] Slightly worried
- [ ] Moderately worried
- [ ] Very worried
- [ ] Extremely worried

My relationship with others

- [ ] Not a worry
- [ ] Slightly worried
- [ ] Moderately worried
- [ ] Very worried
- [ ] Extremely worried

My job

- [ ] Not a worry
- [ ] Slightly worried
- [ ] Moderately worried
- [ ] Very worried
- [ ] Extremely worried

Support I have

- [ ] Not a worry
- [ ] Slightly worried
- [ ] Moderately worried
- [ ] Very worried
- [ ] Extremely worried

Finances

- [ ] Not a worry
- [ ] Slightly worried
- [ ] Moderately worried
- [ ] Very worried
- [ ] Extremely worried

The future

- [ ] Not a worry
- [ ] Slightly worried
- [ ] Moderately worried
- [ ] Very worried
- [ ] Extremely worried

Feeling upset or distressed

- [ ] Not a worry
- [ ] Slightly worried
- [ ] Moderately worried
- [ ] Very worried
- [ ] Extremely worried

Any other concern? Please describe

- [ ] Not a worry
- [ ] Slightly worried
- [ ] Moderately worried
- [ ] Very worried
- [ ] Extremely worried

References

Ahmedzai, S.H. and Shrivastav, S.P. (2000) Breathlessness. *Medicine* **28**, 12–15.

Aitken-Swan, J. and Easson, E.C. (1959) Reactions of cancer patients on being told their diagnosis. *British Medical Journal*, **1**, 779–783.

Aldridge, D. (1992) The needs of individual patients in clinical research. *Advances*, **8**, 58–65.

Andersen, B.L. (1986) Sexual difficulties for women following cancer treatment. In Andersen BL (ed.) *Women with Cancer*. New York: Springer, pp. 257–288.

Andrykowski, M.A., Brady, M.J., and Henslee-Downey, P.J. (1994) Psychosocial factors predictive of survival after allogeneic bone marrow transplantation. *Psychosomatic Medicine*, **56**, 432–439.

Angell, M. (1985) Disease as a reflection of the psyche. *New England Journal of Medicine*, **312**, 1570–1572.

Antoni, M.H. and Goodkin, K. (1988) Host moderator variables in the promotion of cervical neoplasia. I Personality facets. *Journal of Psychosomatic Research*, **32**, 327–338.

Antoni, M.H., Lehman, J.M., Klibourn, K.M., *et al.* (2001) Cognitive-behavioral stress management intervention decreases the prevalence of depression and enhances benefit finding among women under treatment for early-stage breast cancer. *Health Psychology*, **20**, 20–32.

Badger, T.A., Braden, C.J., Longman, A.J., *et al.* (1999) Depression burden, self-help interventions, and social support in women receiving treatment for breast cancer. *Journal of Psychosocial Oncology*, **17**, 17–35.

Baider, L., Cooper, C.L., and De-Nour, A.K. (ed) (1996) *Cancer and the Family*. Chichester: Wiley.

Bartlett, F.C. (1932) *Remembering*. Cambridge: Cambridge University Press.

Barton, R.T. (1965) Life after laryngectomy. *Laryngoscope*, **75**, 1408–1415.

Beck, A.T. (1976) *Cognitive Therapy and the Emotional Disorders*. London: Penguin.

Beck, A.T. (1988) *Love is Never Enough*. New York: Harper Row.

Beck, A.T., Rush, A.J., Shaw, B.F., and Emery, G. (1979) *Cognitive Therapy of Depression*. New York: Guilford Press.

Beck, A.T., Ward, C.H., Mendelson, M., *et al.* (1961) An inventory for measuring depression. *Archives of General Psychiatry*, **4**, 561–571.

Beck, J.S. (1995) *Cognitive Therapy: Basics and Beyond*. New York: Guilford Press.

Beck, R. and Fernandez, E. (1998) Cognitive-behavioral therapy in the treatment of anger: a meta-analysis. *Cognitive Therapy and Research*, **22**, 63–74.

Berglund, G., Bolund, C., Gustaffson, O., *et al.* (1994) A randomised study of a rehabilitation program for cancer patients: The 'starting again' group. *Psycho-Oncology*, **3**, 109–120.

Bloch, S. and Kissane, D.W. (1995) Psychological care and breast cancer. *Lancet*, **346**, 1114.

Bloom, J.R. (1986) Social support and adjustment to breast cancer. In Andersen BL (ed.) *Women with Cancer*. New York: Springer, pp 204–229.

Bloom, J.R. and Spiegel, D. (1984) The relationship of two dimensions of social support to the psychological well-being and social functioning of women with advanced breast cancer. *Social Science & Medicine*, **19**, 831–837.

Bohart, A. (1980) Toward a cognitive theory of catharsis. *Psychotherapy: Theory, Research and Practice*, **17**, 192–201.

Bottomley, A., Hunton, S., Roberts, G., *et al.* (1996) A pilot study of cognitive-behavioural therapy and social support group interventions with newly diagnosed cancer patients. *Journal of Psychosocial Oncology*, **14**, 65–83.

Borkovec, T.D. and Hennings, B.C. (1978) The role of physiological attention-focusing in the relaxation treatment of sleep disturbance, general tension and specific stress reaction. *Behaviour Research and Therapy*, **16**, 17–19.

Borysenko, J., Maurer, S., Stolback, L., *et al.* (1986) Beth Israel Hospital: *Mind/Body Group Program Handbook* (Unpublished manuscript).

Bradford Hill, A. (1961) *Principles of Medical Statistics*. London: The Lancet Ltd.

Brady, S.S. and Helgeson, V.S. (1999) Social support and adjustment to recurrence of breast cancer. *Journal of Psychosocial Oncology*, **17**, 37–55.

Breitbart, W. and Cohen, K.R. (1998) Delirium. In Holland, J.C. (ed.) *Psycho-oncology*. New York: Oxford University Press, pp. 564–575.

Brewin, C.R., Watson, M., McCarthy, S., *et al.* (1998) Intrusive memories and depression in cancer patients. *Behaviour Research and Therapy*, **36**, 1131–1142.

Bruera, E., Miller, L., and McCallion, S. (1990) Cognitive failure in patients with terminal cancer: a prospective longitudinal study. *Psychosocial Aspects of Cancer*, **9**, 308–310.

Buddeberg, C., Wolf, C., and Sieber, M. (1991) Coping strategies and course of disease of breast cancer patients. *Psychotherapy and Psychosomatics*, **55**, 151–157.

Bukberg, J., Penman, G., and Holland, J.C. (1984) Depression in hospitalised cancer patients. *Psychosomatic Medicine*, **46**, 199–212.

Burns, D.D. (1980) *Feeling Good: The New Mood Therapy*. New York: William Morrow.

Burns, D.D. and Auerbach, A. (1996) Therapeutic empathy in cognitive behaviour therapy: does it really make a difference? In Salkovskis, P.M. (ed.) *Frontiers of Cognitive Therapy*. New York: The Guilford Press.

Cain, E.N., Kohorn, E.l., Quinlan, D.M., *et al.* (1986) Psychosocial benefits of a cancer support group. *Cancer*, **57**, 183–189.

Carter, R.E., Carter, C.A., and Prosen, H.A. (1993) Emotional and personality types of breast cancer patients and spouses. *American Journal of Family Therapy*, **20**, 300–309.

Carver, C.S., Pozo, C., Harris, S.D., *et al.* (1993) How coping mediates the effect of optimism on distress: a study of women with early stage breast cancer. *Journal of Personality and Social Psychology*, **65**, 375–390.

Cassileth, B.R., Lusk, E.J., Miller, D.S., *et al.* (1985) Psychological correlates of survival in advanced malignant disease. *New England Journal of Medicine*, **312**, 1551–1555.

Castonguay, L.G., Goldfried, M.R., Wiser, S., *et al.* (1996) Predicting the effect of cognitive therapy for depression: a study of unique and common factors. *Journal of Consulting and Clinical Psychology*, **64**, 497–504.

Cawley, R.H. (1983) The principles of treatment and therapeutic evaluation. In Shepherd, M., Zangwill, O.L. (eds) *General Psychopathology.* Cambridge: Cambridge University Press, pp. 221–243.

Chemtob, C.M., Novaco, R.W., Hamada, R.S., *et al.* (1997) Cognitive-behavioral treatment for severe anger in posttraumatic stress disorder. *Journal of Consulting and Clinical Psychology,* **65,** 184–189.

Clark, D.A. and Steer, R.A. (1996) Empirical status of the cognitive model of anxiety and depression. In Salkovskis PM (ed.) *Frontiers of Cognitive Therapy.* New York: The Guilford Press.

Classen, C., Koopman, C., Angell, K., *et al.* (1996) Coping styles associated with psychological adjustment to advanced breast cancer. *Health Psychology,* **15,** 434–437.

Classen, C., Sephton, S.E., Diamond, S., *et al.* (1998) Studies of life-extending psychosocial interventions. In Holland JC (ed.) *Psycho-oncology.* New York: Oxford University Press, pp. 730–742.

Cochrane, D., Hacker, N.F., Wellisch, D.K., *et al.* (1987) Sexual functioning after treatment for endometrial cancer. *Journal of Psychosocial Oncology,* **5,** 47–61.

Cohn, K.H. (1982) Chemotherapy from an insider's perspective. *Lancet,* **i,** 1006–1009.

Cooper, A. (1982) Disabilities and how to live with them: Hodgkin's disease. *Lancet,* **i,** 612–613.

Coursey, K., Dawson, J.J., and Luce, J.K. (1975) Comparative anxiety levels of cancer patients and family members. *Proceedings of the American Association for Cancer Research,* **16,** 246.

Cox, D.R. (1972) Regression models and life tables. *Journal of the Royal Statistical Society,* **34B,** 187–202.

Crary, W.G. and Crary, G.C. (1974) Emotional crisis and cancer. *Cancer,* **24,** 36–39.

Cunningham, A.J. (1995) Adjuvant psychological therapy for cancer patients: putting it on the same footing as adjunctive medical therapies. *Psycho-Oncology,* **9,** 367–371.

Cunningham, A.J. (1999) Mind-body research in psychooncology: what directions will be most useful? *Advances in Mind-Body Medicine,* **15,** 252–255.

Cunningham, A.J. and Toccom E,K. (1989) A randomized trial of group psychoeducational therapy for cancer patients. *Patient Education Counseling,* **14,** 101–114.

Cunningham, A.J., Lockwood, G.A., and Cunnigham, J.A. (1991) A relationship between self-efficacy and quality of life in cancer patients. *Patient Education and Counselling,* **17,** 71–78.

Cunningham, A.J., Lockwood, G.A., and Edmonds, C.V. (1993) Which cancer patients benefit from a brief, group, coping skills programme? *International Journal of Psychiatry in Medicine,* **23,** 383–398.

Cunningham, A.J., Edmonds, C.V.I., Jenkins, G. *et al.* (1995) A randomised comparison of two forms of brief, group, psychoeducational program for cancer patients: weekly sessions vs a 'weekend intensive.' *International Journal of Psychiatry in Medicine,* **25,** 171–187.

Cunningham, A.J., Edmonds, C.V.I., Jenkins, G.P., *et al.* (1998) A randomised control trial of the effects of group therapy on survival in women with metastatic breast cancer. *Psycho-Oncology,* **7,** 508–517.

Dattilio, F.M. (1997) Family therapy. In R.L. Leahy (ed.) *Practising cognitive therapy: A guide to interventions* Northvale, NJ: Jason Aronson, pp. 409–450.

Dattilio, F.M. and Padesky, C.A. (1990) *Cognitive Therapy with Couples.* Saratosa, FL: Professional Resource Exchange.

Dean, C. and Surtees, P.G. (1995) Do psychological factors predict survival in breast cancer? *Journal of Psychosomatic Research* **13**, 47–66.

de Haes, J.C.J.M., Raatgever, J.W., van den Burg, M.E.L., *et al.* (1987) Evaluation of the quality of life of patients with advanced ovarian cancer treated with combination chemotherapy. In Aaronson, N.K., Beckmann, J. (eds) *The Quality of Life of Cancer Patients.* New York: Raven Press, pp. 215–226.

Deffenbacher, J.L. (1999) Cognitive-behavioral conceptualization and treatment of anger. *Journal of Clinical Psychology,* **55**, 295–309.

Derogatis, L.R., Abeloff, M.D., and Melisaratos, N. (1979) Psychological coping mechanisms and survival time in metastatic breast cancer. *Journal of the American Medical Association,* **249**, 751–757.

Derogatis, L.R. (1983) Psychosocial Adjustment to Illness Scale (PAIS and PAIS—SR). Scoring, procedures and administration manual 1. Baltimore, Clinical Psychometric Research.

Devlin, H.B., Plant, J.A., and Griffin, M. (1971) Aftermath of surgery for ano-rectal cancer. *British Medical Journal,* **3**, 413–418.

Di Clemente, K.J. and Temoshok, L. (1985) Psychological adjustment to having cutaneous malignant melanoma as a predictor of follow-up clinical status. *Psychosomatic Medicine,* **47**, 81.

Drummond, S. (1967) Vocal rehabilitation after laryngectomy. *British Journal of Disorders of Communication,* **2**, 39–44.

Eardley, A., George, W.D., Davis, F., *et al.* (1976) Colostomy: the consequences of surgery. *Clinical Oncology,* **2**, 277–283.

Edelman, S., Lemon, J., Bell, D.R., *et al.* (1999a) Effects of group CBT on the survival time of patients with metastatic breast cancer. *Psycho-Oncology,* **8**, 474–481.

Edelman, S., Bell D.R., and Kidman, A.D. (1999b) A group cognitive-behaviour therapy programme with metastatic breast cancer patients. *Psycho-Oncology,* **8**, 295–305.

Edgar, L., Rosberger, Z., and Nowlis, D. (1992) Coping with cancer during the first year after diagnosis. Assessment and intervention. *Cancer,* **69**, 817–28.

Edmonds, C.V.I., Lockwood, G.A., and Cunningham, A.J. (1999) Psychological response to long term group therapy: a randomized trial with metastatic breast cancer patients. *Psycho-Oncology,* **8**, 74–91.

Eissler, K.R. (1955) *The Psychiatrist and the Dying Patient.* New York: International University Press.

Ell, K., Nishimoto, R., and Morvay, T. (1989) A longitudinal analysis of psychological adaptation among survivors of cancer. *Cancer,* **63**, 406–413.

Elliotson, J. (1848) *Cure of True Cancer with Mesmerism.* London: Walton and Mitchell.

Elsesser, K., van Berkel, M., Sartory, G., *et al.* (1994) The effects of anxiety management training on psychological variables and immune parameters in cancer patients: a pilot study. *Behavioural and Cognitive Psychotherapy,* **22**, 13–23.

Evans, R.L. and Connis, R.T. (1995) Comparison of brief group therapies for depressed cancer patients receiving radiation treatment. *Public Health Reports,* **110**, 306–311.

Fallowfield, L.J., Baum, M., and Maguire, G.P. (1986) Effects of breast conservation on psychological morbidity associated with diagnosis and treatment of early breast cancer. *British Medical Journal,* **293**, 1331–1334.

Faulkner, A., Webb, P., and Maguire, P. (1991) Communication and counseling skills: educating health professionals working in cancer and palliative care. *Patient Education and Counseling*, **18**, 3–7.

Fawzy, F.I. (1994) The benefits of a short-term group intervention for cancer patients. *Advances*, **10**, 17–19.

Fawzy, F.I. and Fawzy, N.W. (1994) A structured psychosocial intervention for cancer patients. *General Hospital Psychiatry*, **16**, 149–192.

Fawzy, F.I., Kemeny, M.E., Fawzy, N.W., *et al.* (1990a) A structured psychiatric intervention for cancer patients: I changes over times in methods of coping and affective disturbance. *Archives of General Psychiatry*, **47**, 720–725.

Fawzy, F.I., Kemeny, M.E., Fawzy, N.W., *et al.* (1990b) A structured psychiatric intervention for cancer patients. II Changes over time in immunological measures. *Archives of General Psychiatry*, **47**, 729–735.

Fawzy, F.I., Fawzy, N.W., Hyun, C.S., *et al.* (1993) Malignant melanoma: effects of an early structured psychiatric intervention, coping, and affective state on recurrence and survival 6 years later. *Archives of General Psychiatry*, **50**, 681–689.

Fawzy, F.I., Fawzy, N.W., and Wheeler, J.G. (1996) A post-hoc comparison of the efficiency of a psychoeducational intervention for melanoma patients delivered in group versus individual formats: an analysis of data from two studies. *Psycho-Oncology*, **5**, 81–89.

Feigin, R., Greenberg, A., Ras, H., *et al.* (2000) The psychosocial experience of women treated for breast cancer by highdose chemotherapy supported by autologous stem-cell transplant: a qualitative analysis of support groups. *Psycho-Oncology*, **9**, 57–68.

Feinstein, A.D. (1983) Psychological interventions in the treatment of cancer. *Clinical Psychology Review*, **3**, 1–14.

Fennell, M.J.V. and Teasdale, J.D. (1987) Cognitive therapy for depression: individual differences and the process of change. *Cognitive Therapy and Research*, **11**, 253–271.

Fennell, M.J.V., Teasdale, J.D., Jones, S., *et al.* (1987) Distraction in neurotic and endogenous depression: an investigation of negative thinking in major depressive disorders. *Psychological Medicine*, **17**, 441–452.

Fernandez-Ballesteros, R., Ruiz, M.A., and Garde, S. (1998) Emotional expression in healthy women and those with breast cancer. *British Journal of Health Psychology*, **3**, 41–50.

Fichten, K.S. (1986) Self – other and situation-referant automatic thoughts: interaction between people who have a physical disability and those who do not. *Cognitive Therapy and Research*, **10**, 571–587.

Finlay, I.G. (2000) Palliative care: an introduction. *Medicine*, **28**, 1.

Fiore, N. (1979) Fighting cancer—one patient's perspective. *New England Journal of Medicine*, **300**, 284–289.

Fiore, N.A. (1984) *The Road back to Health*. New York: Bantam Books.

Folkman, S. (1997) Positive psychological states and coping with severe stress. *Social Science and Medicine*, **45**, 1207–1221.

Folkman, S. and Greer, S. (2000) Promoting psychological well-being in the face of serious illness: when theory, research and practice inform each other. *Psycho-Oncology*, **9**, 11–19.

Fobair, P., Hoppe, R.J., Bloom, J., *et al.* (1986) Psychosocial problems among survivors of Hodgkin's disease. *Journal of Clinical Oncology*, **4**, 805–814.

Ford, M.F., Jones, M., Scannell, T., *et al.* (1990) Is group psychotherapy feasible for oncology outpatient attenders on the basis of psychological morbidity? *British Journal of Cancer*, **62**, 624–626.

Fox, B.H. (1998a) A hypothesis about Spiegel *et al.*'s 1989 paper on psychosocial intervention and breast cancer survival. *Psycho-Oncology*, **7**, 361–370.

Fox, B.H. (1998b) Rejoinder to Spiegel *et al. Psycho-Oncology*, **7**, 518–519.

Fox, B.H. (1999) Clarification regarding comments about a hypothesis. *Psycho-Oncology*, **8**, 366–367.

Frank, J.D. (1971) Therapeutic factors in psychotherapy. *American Journal of Psychotherapy*, **25**, 350–361.

Freud, S. (1953) Thoughts for the time on war and death (ii). In Strachey, J. (ed.) *The Complete Psychological Works* vol XIV. London: Hogarth, p 289.

Fuller, S. and Swenson, C.H. (1993) Marital and quality of life among cancer patients and their spouses. *Journal of Psychosocial Oncology*, **10**, 41–56.

Girgis, A. and Sanson-Fisher, R.W. (1998) Breaking bad news. 1: Current best advice for clinicians. *Behavioral Medicine*, **24**, 53–59.

Goodkin, K., Antoni, M.H., and Blaney, P.H. (1986) Stress and hopelessness in the promotion of cervical intraepithelial neoplasia to invasive squamous cell carcinoma of the cervix. *Journal of Psychosomatic Research*, **30**, 67–76.

Goodwin, P.J., Leszcz, M., Koopman, J., *et al.* (1996) Randomized trial of group psycho-social support in metastatic breast cancer: the BEST (Breast Expressive-Supportive Therapy) study. *Cancer Treatment Reviews*, **22** (Suppl A), 91–96.

Goodwin, P.J., Pritchard, K.I., and Spiegel, D. (1999) The Fox guarding the clinical trial: internal vs external validity in randomized studies. *Psycho-Oncology*, **8**, 275.

Grandi, S., Fava, G.A., Cunsolo, A., *et al.* (1987) Major depression associated with mastectomy. *Medical Science Research*, **15** (5–8), Mar–Apr 1987, 283–284.

Greenberg, L.S. and Safran, J.D. (1987) *Emotion in Psychotherapy.* New York: Guilford.

Greenberg, D.B., Sawicka, J., Eisenthal, S., *et al.* (1992) Fatigue syndrome due to localized radiation. *Journal of Pain and Symptom Management*, **7**, 38–45.

Greer, S. (1985) Cancer: Psychiatric Aspects. In Granville Grossman K. (ed.) *Recent Advances in Clinical Psychiatry*. Edinburgh: Churchill-Livingstone.

Greer, S. (1995) The psychological toll of cancer. In Horwich, A. (ed.) *Oncology*. London: Chapman and Hall, pp. 189–198.

Greer, S. (1999) Mind-body research in psychooncology. *Advances in Mind–Body Medicine*, **15**, 236–244.

Greer, S. and Burgess, C. (1987) A self-esteem measure for patients with cancer. *Psychology and Health*, **1**, 327–340.

Greer, S. and Morris, T. (1975) Psychological attributes of women who develop breast cancer: a controlled study. *Journal of Psychosomatic Research*, **19**, 147–153.

Greer, S. and Watson, M. (1987) Mental adjustment to cancer: its measurement and prognostic importance. *Cancer Surveys*, **6**, 439–453.

Greer, S., Morris, T., Pettingale, K.W., *et al.* (1990) Psychological response to breast cancer and 15 year outcome. *Lancet*, **i**, 49–50.

Greer, S., Moorey, S., Baruch, J.D.R., *et al.* (1992) Adjuvant psychological therapy for patients with cancer: a prospective randomised trial. *British Medical Journal*, **304**, 675–680.

Harrison, J., Maguire, P., Ibbotson, T., *et al.* (1994) Concerns, confiding and psychiatric disorder in newly diagnosed cancer patients: a descriptive study. *Psycho-oncology*, **3**, 173–179.

Helgeson, V.S. and Cohen, S. (1996) Social support and adjustment to cancer: reconciling descriptive, correlational, and intervention research. *Health Psychology*, **15**, 135–148.

Helgeson, V.S. and Taylor, S.E. (1993) Social comparisons and adjustment among cardiac patients. *Journal of Applied Social Psychology*, **23**, 1171–1195.

Heinrich, R.L. and Schag, C.C. (1985) Stress and activity management group treatment for cancer patients and spouses. *Journal of Counseling and Clinical Psychology*, **53**, 439–446.

Hilton, B.A. (1994) Family communication patterns in coping with early breast cancer. *Western Journal of Nursing Research*, **16**, 366–388.

Hinton, J. (1967) *Dying*. London: Penguin.

Hinton, J. (1981) Sharing or witholding awareness of dying between husband and wife. *Journal of Psychosomatic Research*, **25**, 337–343.

Hinton, J. (1994) Which patients with terminal care are admitted from home care? *Palliative Medicine*, **8**, 197–210.

Hislop, G.T., Waxler, N.E., Coldman, J., *et al.* (1987) The prognostic significance of psychosocial factors in women with breast cancer. *Journal of Chronic Diseases*, **40**, 729–735.

Holland, J.C., Korzun, A.H., Tross, S., *et al.* (1986) Psychosocial factors and disease-free survival in Stage II breast carcinoma. *Proceedings American Society of Clinical Oncology*, **5**, 237 (Abstract).

Holland, J.C. and Marchini, I.A. (1998) International psycho-oncology. In Holland JC (ed.) *Psycho-Oncology*. New York: Oxford University Press, pp. 1165–1169.

Horowitz, M.J. (1986) *Stress Response Syndromes*. Northvale, London: Aronson.

Horwich, A. (1995) Testicular cancer. In Horwich A (ed.) *Oncology*. London: Chapman and Hall, pp. 485–498.

Hughes, J.E. (1985) Depressive illness and lung cancer. II. Follow-up of inoperable patients. *European Journal of Surgical Oncology*, **11**, 21–24.

Hughes, J.E. (1987) Psychological and social consequences of cancer. *Cancer Surveys*, **6**, 455–475.

Ilnyckyj, A., Farber, J., Cheang, M.C., *et al.* (1994) A randomized controlled trial of psychotherapeutic intervention in cancer patients. *Annals Royal College of Physicians and Surgeons*, Canada, **27**, 93–96.

Irvine, D., Brown, B., Crooks, D., *et al.* (1991) Psychosocial adjustment of women with breast cancer. *Cancer*, **67**, 1097–1117.

Irving, L.M., Snyder, C.R., and Crowson, J.J. (1998) Hope and coping with cancer by college women. *Journal of Personality*, **66**, 195–214.

Jamison, R.N., Burnish, T.G., and Wallston, K.A. (1987) Psychogenic factors in predicting survival of breast cancer patients. *Journal of Clinical Oncology*, **5**, 768–772.

Janoff-Bulman, R. (1992) *Shattered Assumptions: Towards a new psychology of trauma.* New York: Free Press.

Janoff-Bulman, R. (1999) Rebuilding shattered assumptions after traumatic life events: coping processes and outcomes. In Snyder, C.R. (ed.) *Coping: The Psychology of What Works.* Oxford: Oxford University Press.

Jensen, M.R. (1987) Psychobiological factors predicting the course of cancer. *Journal of Personality,* **55,** 329–342.

Johnson, J. (1982) The effects of a patient education course on patients with a chronic illness. *Cancer Nurse,* April: 117–123.

Kabat-Zinn, J., Lipworth, L., and Burney, R. (1985) The clinical use of mindfulness meditation for the self-regulation of chronic pain. *Journal of Behavioral Medicine,* **8,** 163–190.

Kabat-Zinn, J., Massion, A.O., Kristeller, J., *et al.* (1992) Effectiveness of a meditation-based stress reduction program in the treatment of anxiety disorders. *American Journal of Psychiatry,* **149,** 936–943.

Kausar, R. and Akram, M. (1998) Cognitive appraisal and coping of patients with terminal versus nonterminal diseases. *Journal of Behavioural Sciences,* **9,** 13–28.

Kingdon, D.G. and Turkington, D. (1994) *Cognitive Behavioural Therapy of Schizophrenia.* Guilford: Psychology Press.

Kissane, D.W., Bloch, S., Miach, P., *et al.* (1997) Cognitive-existential group therapy for patients with primary breast cancer—techniques and themes. *Psycho-Oncology,* **6,** 25–33.

Kornblith, A.B., Anderson, J., and Cella, D.F. (1992) Hodgkin's disease survivors at increased risk for problems in psychosocial adaptation. *Cancer,* **70,** 2214–2224.

Kovacs, M. and Beck, A.T. (1978) Maladaptive cognitive structures in depression. *American Journal of Psychiatry,* **135,** 525–533.

Kuipers, E., Garety, P., Fowler, D., *et al.* (1997) London-East Anglia randomised controlled trial of cognitive behavioural therapy for psychosis. I: effects of the treatment phase. *British Journal of Psychiatry,* **171,** 319–327.

Lakein, A. (1973) *How to Get Control of Your Time and Your Life.* New York: New American Library.

Lazarus, R.S. and Folkman, S. (1984) *Stress, Appraisal and Coping.* New York: Springer.

Levine, P.M., Silberfarb, P.M., and Lipowski, Z.J. (1978) Mental disorders in cancer patients. *Cancer,* **42,** 1385–1391.

Levy, S.M., Lee, J., Bagley, C., *et al.* (1988) Survival hazards analysis in first recurrent breast cancer patients: seven-year follow-up. *Psychosomatic Medicine,* **50,** 520–528.

Lewis, A. (1958) Between guesswork and certainty in psychiatry. *Lancet,* **i,** 171–175 and 227–230.

Lewis, W.A. and Bucher, A.M. (1992) Anger, catharsis, the reformulated frustration-aggression hypothesis, and health consequences. *Psychotherapy,* **29,** 385–392.

Lichtman, R.R. and Taylor, S.E. (1986) Close relationships and the female cancer patient. In Andersen, B.L. (ed.) *Women with Cancer.* New York: Springer, pp. 233–256.

Lichtman, R.R., Taylor, S.E., Wood, J.V., *et al.* (1985) Relations with children after breast cancer: the mother-daughter relationship at risk. *Journal of Psychosocial Oncology,* **2,** 1–19.

Liese, B.S. and Larson, M.W. (1995) Coping with life-threatening illness: a cognitive therapy perspective. *Journal of Cognitive Psychotherapy*, **9**, 19–34.

Linn, M.W., Linn, B.S., and Harris, R. (1982) Effects of counselling for late stage cancer patients. Cancer, **49**, 1048–1055.

Lloyd, G.G. (1979) Psychological stress and coping mechanisms in patients with cancer. In Stoll, B.A. (ed.) *Mind and Cancer Prognosis*. Chichester: John Wiley, pp. 47–59.

Lloyd-Williams, M. and Friedman, T. (1999) Depression in terminally ill patients. *American Journal of Hospice Palliative Care*, **16**, 704.

Lumley, M.A., Kelley, J.E., and Leissen, J.C.C. (1997) Health effects of emotional disclosure in rheumatoid arthritis patients. *Health Psychology*, **16**, 331–340.

McIntosh, J. (1974) Process of communication, information seeking and control associated with cancer. *Social Science and Medicine*, **8**,167–187.

McNair, D., Lorr, M., and Droppleman, L. (1970) *Manual for Profile of Mood States*. San Diego: education and Industrial Testing Service.

Magee, B. (1997) *Confessions of a Philosopher*. London: Weidenfeld and Nicholson, pp. 214–215.

Maguire, G.P., Lee, E.G., Bevington, D.J., *et al.* (1978) Psychiatric problems in the first year after mastectomy. *British Medical Journal*, **1**, 963–965.

Maguire, G.P., Tait, A., Brooke, M., *et al.* (1980) Psychiatric morbidity and physical toxicity associated with adjuvant chemotherapy and mastectomy. *British Medical Journal*, **281**, 1179–1180.

Maguire, P. (1979) The will to live in the cancer patient. In Stoll, B.A. (ed.) *Mind and Cancer Prognosis*. Chichester: Wiley, pp. 169–182.

Masters, W.H. and Johnson, V.E. (1970) *Human Sexual Inadequacy*. Boston: Little, Brown.

Meichenbaum, D. (1977) Cognitive-behaviour Modification: an Integrative Approach. New York: Plenum Press.

Meichenbaum, D. (1985) *Stress Inoculation Training*. Oxford: Pergamon Press.

Meyer, T.J. and Mark, M.M. (1995) Effects of psychosocial interventions with adult cancer patients: a meta-analysis of randomized experiments. *Health Psychology*, **14**, 101–108.

Middleboe, T., Ovesen, L., Mortensen, E., *et al.* (1995) The relationship between self-reported general health and observed depression and anxiety in cancer patients during chemotherapy. *Nordic Journal of Psychiatry*, **49**, 25–31.

Miller, J.J., Fletcher, K., and Kabat-Zinn, J. (1995) Three-year follow-up and clinical implications of a mindfulness meditation-based stress reduction intervention in the treatment of anxiety disorders. *General Hospital Psychiatry*, **17**, 192–200.

Mitchell, G.W. and Glickman, A.S. (1977) Cancer patients: knowledge and attitudes. *Cancer*, **40**, 61–66.

Montgomery, C., Lydon, A., and Lloyd, K. (1999) Psychological distress among cancer patients and informed consent. *Journal of Psychosomatic Research*, **46**, 241–245.

Moorey, S. (1996) When bad things happen to rational people: cognitive therapy in adverse life situations. In Salkovskis, P. (ed.) *Frontiers of Cognitive Therapy*. New York: Guilford Press.

Moorey, S. and Greer, S. (1989) *Psychological Therapy for Patients with Cancer*. Oxford: Heinemann Medical Book.

Moorey, S., Greer, S., Watson, M., *et al.* (1991) The factor structure and factor stability of the Hospital Anxiety and Depression Scale in patients with cancer. *British Journal of Psychiatry*, **158**, 255–259.

Moorey, S., Greer, S., Watson, M., *et al.* (1994) Adjuvant psychological therapy for patients with cancer: outcome at one year. *Psycho-oncology*, **3**, 39–46.

Moorey, S., Greer, S., Bliss, J., *et al.* (1998) A comparison of adjuvant psychological therapy and supportive counselling in patients with cancer. *Psycho-Oncology*, **7**, 218–228.

Moorey, S., Frampton, M., and Greer, S. (in press) The Cancer Coping Questionnaire: a self-rating scale for measuring the impact of adjuvant psychological therapy on coping behaviour *Submitted to Psycho-oncology*.

Morris, T., Greer, H.S., and White, P. (1977) Psychological and social adjustment to mastectomy: a two-year follow-up study. *Cancer*, **77**, 2381–2387.

Morris, T., Blake, S., and Buckley, M. (1985) Development of a method of rating for cognitive responses to a diagnosis of cancer. *Social Science and Medicine*, **20**, 795–802.

Morris, T., Pettingale, K., and Haybittle, J. (1992) Psychological response to cancer diagnosis and disease outcome in patients with breast cancer and lymphoma. *Psycho-Oncology*, 105–114.

Morize, V., Nguyen, D.T., Lorente, C., *et al.* (1999) Descriptive epidemiological survey on a given day in all palliative care patients hospitalized in a French University Hospital. *Palliative Medicine*, **13**, 105–117.

Morrow, G.R., Asbury, R., Hammon, S., *et al.* (1992) Comparing the effectiveness of behavioral treatment for chemotherapy-induced nausea and vomiting when administered by oncologists, oncology nurses, and clinical psychologists. *Health Psychology*, **11**, 250–256.

Moynihan, C. (1987) Testicular cancer: the psychosocial problems of patient and their relatives. *Cancer Surveys*, **6**, 477–510.

Moynihan, C., Bliss, J.M., Davidson, J., *et al.* (1998) Evaluation of Adjuvant Psychological Therapy in patients with testicular cancer: a randomised trial. *British Medical Journal*, **316**, 429–435.

Northouse, L.L., Dorris, G., and Charron-Moore, C. (1996) Factors affectings couple's adjustment to recurrent breast cancer. *Social Science and Medicine*, **41**, 69–76.

Northouse, L.L., Templin, T., Mood, D., *et al.* (1998) Couples' adjustment to breast cancer and benign breast disease: a longitudinal analysis. *Psycho-Oncology*, **7**, 37–48.

Novaco, R.W. (1976) The functions and regulation of the arousal of anger. *American Journal of Psychiatry*, **133**, 1124–1128.

Novaco, R.W. (1995) Clinical problems of anger and its assessment and regulation through a stress coping skills approach. In O'Donohue W *et al.* (eds) *Handbook of psychological skills training: Clinical techniques and applications*. Boston: Allyn and Bacon.

Novaco, R.W. and Chemtob, C.M. (1998) Anger and trauma: conceptualization, assessment, and treatment. In Follette, V.M., Ruzek, J.I., *et al.* (eds) *Cognitive-behavioral therapies for trauma*. New York: The Guilford Press.

Oken, D. (1961) What to tell cancer patients: a study of medical attitudes. *Journal of the American Medical Association*, **175**, 1120–1128.

Osborne, R.H., Elsworth, G.R., Kissane, D.W., *et al.* (1999) The Mental Adjustment to Cancer (MAC) Scale: replication and refinement in 632 breast cancer patients. *Psychological Medicine,* **29,** 1335–1345.

Parle, M., Maguire, P., and Heaven, C. (1997) The development of a training model to improve health professionals' skills, self-efficacy and outcome expectancies when communicating with cancer patients. *Social Science and Medicine,* **44,** 231–240.

Parloff, M.B., Waskow, I.E., and Wolfe, B.E. (1978) Research on therapist variables in relation to process and outcome research. In Garfield, S.L., Bergin, A .(eds) *Handbook of Psychotherapy and Behaviour Change: an Empirical Analysis,* 2nd edn. New York: John Wiley.

Peck, A. (1972) Emotional reactions to having cancer. *American Journal of Roentgenology, Radium Therapy and Nuclear Medicine,* **114,** 591–599.

Perloff, L.S. (1983) Perceptions of vulnerability to victimisation. *Journal of Social Issues,* **39,** 41–61.

Perloff, L.S. (1987) Illusions of invulnerability. In Snyder, C.R., Ford, C.E. (eds) *Coping with Negative Life Events.* New York: Plenum Press.

Persons, J.B., Davidson, J., and Tompkins, M.A. (2001) *Essential Components of Cognitive-Behavior Therapy for Depression.* Washington DC: American Psychological Association.

Pettingale, K.W., Philalethis, A., Tee, D.E.H., *et al.* (1981) The biological correlates of psychological responses to cancer. *Journal of Psychosomatic Research,* **25,** 453–458.

Pettingale, K.W., Burgess, C., and Greer, S. (1988) Psychological response to cancer diagnosis. I. Correlations with prognostic variables. *Journal of Psychosomatic Research,* **32,** 255–261.

Phillips, D.P. and Smith, D.G. (1990) Postponement of death until symbolically meaningful occasions. *Journal ofAmerican Medical Association,* **263,** 1947–1951.

Pistrang, N. and Barker, C. (1995) The partner relationship in psychological response to breast cancer. *Social Science and Medicine,* **40,** 789–797.

Ratcliffe, M.A., Dawson, A.A., and Walker, L.G. (1995) Eysenck Personality Inventory L-scores in patients with Hodgkin's disease and non-Hodgkin's lymphoma. *Psycho-Oncology,* **4,** 39–45.

Rieker, P.P., Edbril, S.D., and Garnick, M.B. (1985) Curative testis cancer therapy: psychosocial sequelae. *Journal of Clinical Oncology,* **3,** 1117–1126.

Renneker, R.E. (1982) Cancer and psychotherapy. In Goldberg JG (ed) *Psychotherapeutic Treatment of Cancer Patients.* New York: Free Press.

Richardson, J.L., Shelton, D.R., Krailo, M., *et al.* (1990) The effect of compliance with treatment on survival among patients with hematologic malignancies. *Journal of Clinical Oncology,* **8,** 356–364.

Ringdal, G.I. (1995) Correlates of hopelessness in cancer patients. *Journal of Psychosocial Oncology,* **13,** 47–66.

Rodrigue, J.R. and Park, T.L. (1996) General and illness-specific adjustment to cancer: relationship to marital status and marital quality. *Journal of Psychosomatic Research,* **40,** 29–36.

Salkovskis, P.M. and Warwick, N.M.C. (1986) Morbid preoccupations, health anxiety and reassurance: a cognitive-behavioural approach to hypochondriasis, *Behaviour Research and Therapy,* **24,** 597–602.

Schmale, A.H., Morrow, G.R., Davis, A., *et al.* (1982) Pretreatment behaviour profiles associated with subsequent psychosocial adjustment in radiation therapy patients: a prospective study. *International Journal of Psychiatry in Medicine*, **12**, 187–195.

Schover, L.R. (1998) Sexual dysfunction. In Holland, J.C. (ed.) *Psycho-Oncology*. New York, Oxford University Press, pp. 494–499.

Selawry, O. (1979) The individual and the median. In Stoll, B.A. (ed.) *Mind and Cancer Prognosis*. Chichester: Wiley, pp. 39–43.

Sellick, S.M. and Crooks, D.L. (1999) Depression and cancer: an appraisal of the literature for prevalence, detection, and practice guideline development for psychological interventions. *Psycho-Oncology*, **8**, 315–333.

Servaes, P., Vingerhoets, A.J.J.M., Vreugdenhill, G., *et al.* (1999) Inhibition of emotional expression in breast cancer patients. *Behavioral Medicine*, **25**, 23–27.

Sheard, T. and Maguire (1999) The effect of psychological interventions on anxiety and depression in cancer patients: results of two meta-analyses. *British Journal of Cancer*, **80**, 1770–1780.

Silberfarb, P.M. and Greer, S. (1982) Psychological concomitants of cancer: clinical aspects. *American Journal of Psychotherapy*, **36**, 470–478.

Simonton, S. and Sherman, A. (2000) An integrated model of group treatment for cancer patients. *International Journal of Group Psychotherapy*, **50**, 487–506.

Simonton, S., Simonton, O.C., and Creighton, J.C. (1978) *Getting Well Again*. New York: Bantam Books.

Smyth, J.M. and Pennebaker, J.W. (1999) Sharing one's story: translating emotional experiences into words as a coping tool. In Snyder, C.R. (ed.) *Coping: The Psychology of What Works*. New York: Oxford University Press.

Speca, M. (1999) Rejoinder to Fox. *Psycho-Oncology*, **8**, 276.

Speca, M., Carlson, L.E., Goodey, E., and Angen, M. (2000) A randomized, wait-list controlled clinical trial: the effect of a mindfulness meditation-based stress reduction program on mood and symptoms of stress in cancer outpatients. *Psychosomatic Medicine*, **62**, 613–622.

Speice, J., Harkness, J., Laneri, H., *et al.* (2000) Involving family members in cancer care: focus group considerations of patients and oncological providers. *Psycho-Oncology*, **9**, 101–112.

Spiegel, D. (1985) Psychosocial interventions with cancer patients. *Journal of Psychosocial Oncology*, **3**, 83–95.

Spiegel, D. and Spira, J. (1991) *Supportive-Expressive Group Therapy: A Treatment Manual of Psychosocial Intervention for Women with Recurrent Breast Cancer*. Stanford, CA.: Stanford University School of Medicine

Spiegel, D., Bloom, J.R., and Yalom, I.D. (1981) Group support for patients with metastatic cancer. *Archives of General Psychiatry*, **38**, 527–533.

Spiegel, D., Bloom, J.R., Kraemer, H.C., *et al.* (1989) Effect of psychosocial treatment on survival of patients with metastatic breast cancer. *Lancet*, **ii**, 888–891.

Spiegel, D., Kraemer, H.C., and Bloom, J.R. (1998) A tale of two methods: randomisation versus matching trials in clinical research. *Psycho-Oncology*, **7**, 371–375.

Spiegel, D., Morrow, G.R., Classen, C., *et al.* (1999) Group therapy for recently diagnosed breast cancer patients: a multicenter feasibility study. *Psycho-Oncology*, **8**, 482–483.

Spielberger, C.D., Gorsuch, R.L., and Lushene, R.F. (1970) *Manual for the State Trait Anxiety Inventory*. Palo Alto, CA: Consulting Psychologists Press.

Spira, J.L. (1998) Group therapies. In Holland, J.C. (ed.) *Psycho-Oncology*, New York: Oxford University Press, pp. 701–716.

Stanton, A.L., Danoff-burg, S., Cameron, C., *et al.* (2000a) Emotionally expressive coping predicts psychological and physical adjustment to breast cancer. *Journal of Consulting and Clinical Psychology*, **68**, 875–882.

Stanton, A.L., Kirk, S.B., Cameron, C.L., *et al.* (2000b) Coping through emotional approach: scale construction and validation. *Health Psychology*, **12**, 16–23.

Tarrier, N. and Maguire, P. (1984) Treatment of psychological distress following mastectomy: an initial report. *Behaviour Research and Therapy*, **22**, 81–84.

Taylor, S.E. and Armor, D.A. (1996) Positive illusions and coping with adversity. *Journal of Personality*, **64**, 873–898.

Taylor, S.E., Lichtman, R.R., and Wood, J.V. (1984) Attributions, beliefs about control and adjustment to breast cancer. *Journal of Personality and Social Psychology*, **46**, 489–502.

Taylor, S.E., Kemeny, M.E., Aspinwall, L.G. ,*et al.* (1993) Optimism, coping, psychological distress, and high-risk sexual behavior among men at risk for acquired immunodeficiency syndrome (AIDS). *Journal of Personality and Social Psychology*, **63**, 460–473.

Taylor, S.E., Kemeny, M.E., Reed, G.M., *et al.* (2000) Psychological resources, positive illusions, and health. *American Psychologist*, **55**, 99–109.

Teasdale, J.D. (1983) Change in cognition during depression—psychopathological implications: discussion paper. *Journal of the Royal Society of Medicine*, **76**, 1038–1044.

Telch, C.F. and Telch, M.J. (1986) Group coping skills instruction and supportive group therapy for cancer patients: a comparison of strategies. *Journal of Consulting and Clinical Psychology*, **34**, 802–808.

Temoshok, L. (1985) Biopsychosocial studies on cutaneous malignant melanoma: psychosocial factors associated with progression, psychophysiology and tumor-host response. *Social Science and Medicine*, **20**, 833–840.

Tennen, H. and Afflleck, G. (1999) Finding benefits in adversity. In Snyder, C.R. (ed.) *Coping: The Psychology of What Works*. Oxford: Oxford University Press.

Teno, J.M. (1999) Lessons learned and not learned from the SUPPORT project. *Palliative Medicine*, **13**, 91–93.

Thomas, C., Turner, P., and Madden, F. (1988) Coping and the outcome of stoma surgery. *Journal of Psychosomatic Research*, **4**, 457–467.

Trillin, A.S. (1981) Of dragons and garden peas: a cancer patient talks to doctors. *New England Journal of Medicine*, **304**, 699–701.

Tross, S., Hendon, J., Korzun, A., *et al.* (1996) Psychological symptoms and disease-free and overall survival in women with 11 breast cancer and leukaemia group B. *Journal of the National Cancer Institute*, **88**, 661–667.

Turk, D.C. and Fernandez, E. (1991) Pain: a cognitive-behavioural perspective. In Watson, M. (ed.) *Cancer patient care: Psychosocial treatment methods*. New York: Cambridge University Press.

Turner, R. (1995) Principles of palliative care. In Horwich, A. (ed.) *Oncology*. London: Chapman and Hall, pp. 199–211.

Vachon, M.L.S., Freedman, K., Formo, A., *et al.* (1977) The final illness in cancer: the widow's perspective. *Canadian Medical Association Journal*, **117**, 1151–1154.

Van Herringen, C., Van Moffaert, M., and de Cuypere, G. (1990) Depression after surgery for breast cancer: comparison of mastectomy and lumpectomy. *Psychotherapy and Psychosomatics*, **51**, 175–179.

von Eschenbach, A.C. (1986) Sexual dysfunction following therapy for cancer of the prostate, testis and penis. In Vaeth J M (ed.). Body Image, *Self-Esteem and Sexuality in Cancer Patients.* Basel: Karger, pp. 48–55.

Watson, M. (1993) Anticipatory nausea and vomiting: broadening the scope of psychological treatments. *Support-Care-Cancer*, **1**, 171–177.

Watson, M. and Greer, S. (1998) Coping and personality. In Holland, J.C. (ed.) *Psycho-Oncology.* New York: Oxford University Press, pp. 81–98.

Watson, M. and Marvell, C. (1992) Anticipatory nausea and vomiting among cancer patients: a review. *Psychology and Health*, **6**, 97–106.

Watson, M,, Pettingale, K.W., and Greer, S. (1984) Emotional control and autonomic arousal in breast cancer patients. *Journal of Psychosomatic Research*, **28**, 467–474.

Watson, M., Greer, S., Young, J., *et al.* (1988) Development of a questionnaire measure of adjustment to cancer: the MAC scale. *Psychological Medicine*, **18**, 203–209.

Watson, M., Greer, S., Pruyn, J., *et al.* (1990) Locus of control and adjustment to cancer. *Psychological Reports*, **66**, 39–48.

Watson, M., Law, M., dos Santos, M., *et al.* (1994) The Mini-MAC: further development of the mental adjustment to cancer scale. *Journal of Psychosocial Oncology*, **12**, 33–46.

Watson, M., Haviland, J.S., Greer, S., *et al.* (1999) Influence of psychological response on survival in breast cancer: a population-based cohort study. *Lancet*, **354**, 1331–1336.

Weinstein, M. (1974) Allocation of subjects in medical experiments. *New England Journal of Medicine*, **291**, 1278–1285.

Weinstein, N.D. (1980) Unrealistic optimism about future life events. *Journal of Personality and Social Psychology*, **39**, 806–820.

Weinstein, N.D. and Lachendro, E. (1982) Egocentrism as a source of unrealistic optimism. *Personality and Social Psychology Bulletin*, **8**, 195–200.

Weisman, A.D. and Worden, J.W. (1977) *Coping and Vulnerability in Cancer Patients.* Boston:Massachusetts General Hospital.

Weisman, A.D., Worden, J.W., and Sobel, H.J. (1980) Psychosocial screening and intervention with cancer patients. *Project Omega*, Boston: Harvard Medical School.

Wellisch, D.K., Gritz, E.R., Schain, W., *et al.* (1992) Psychological functioning of daughters of breast cancer patients. Part II. Characterizing the distressed daughter of the breast cancer patient. *Psychosomatics*, **33**, 171–179.

Wells, A. (1997) *Cognitive Therapy of Anxiety Disorders.* Chichester: Wiley.

Wells, A. (2000) *Emotional disorders and metacognition: Innovative cognitive therapy.* Chichester: Wiley.

Wessely, S., Rose, S., and Bisson, J. (2000) Brief psychological interventions ("debriefing") for trauma-related symptoms and the prevention of post traumatic stress disorder. *Cochrane Database of Systematic Reviews.*

White, C.A. (2001) *Cognitive Behaviour Therapy for Chronic Medical Problems: a Guide to Assessment and Treatment in Practice.* Cichester: Wiley.

Williams, C. (1997) A cognitive model of dysfunctional illness behaviour. *British Journal of Health Psychology*, **2**, 153–165.

Williams, N.L. and Johnston, D. (1983) The quality of life after rectal excision for low rectal cancer. *British Journal of Surgery*, **70**, 460–462.

Winer, E.P., Lindley, C., Hardee, M., *et al.* (1999) Quality of life in patients surviving at least 12 months following high dose chemotherapy with autologous bone marrow support. *Psycho-Oncology*, **8**, 167–176.

Wirsching, M., Druner, H.U., and Herrman, C. (1975) Results of psychosocial adjustment to long-term colostomy. *Psychotherapy and Psychosomatics*, **26**, 245–256.

Wirsching, M., Georg, W., Hoffmann, F., *et al.* (1988) Psychosocial factors influencing health development in breast cancer and mastopathia. In Cooper, C.L. (ed.) *Stress and Breast Cancer*. Wiley: Chichester, pp. 99–107.

Wiser, S. and Arnow, B. (2001) Emotional experiencing: to facilitate or regulate? *Journal of Clinical Psychology*, **57**, 157–168.

Wiser, S. and Goldfried, M.R. (1998) Therapist interventions and client emotional experiencing in expert psychodynamic-interpersonal and cognitive-behavioral therapies. *Journal of Consulting and Clinical Psychology*, **66**, 634–640.

Worden, J.W., Johnston, L.C., and Harrison, R.H. (1974) Survival quotient as a method of investigating psychosocial aspects of cancer survival. *Psychological Reports*, **35**, 719–726.

Worden, J.W. and Weisman, A.D. (1984) Preventive psychosocial intervention with newly diagnosed cancer patients. *General Hospital Psychiatry*, **6**, 243–249.

Wortman, C.B. and Dunkel-Schetter, C. (1979) Interpersonal relationships and cancer: a theoretical analysis. *Journal of Social Issues*, **35**, 120–155.

World Health Organisation (1990) *Cancer Pain Relief and Palliative Care*. Geneva: WHO.

Zabora, J.R., Smith-Wilson, R., Fetting, J.H., *et al.* (1990) An efficient method for the psychosocial screening of cancer patients. *Psychosomatics*, **31**, 192–196.

Zahlis, E.H. and Lewis, F.M. (1998) Mothers' stories of the school-age child's experience with the mother's breast cancer. *Journal of Psychosocial Oncology*, **16**, 25–43.

Zigmond, A.S. and Snaith, R.P. (1983) The Hospital Anxiety and Depression Scale. *Acta Psychiatrica Scandinavia*, **67**, 361–370.

Zucchero, R.A. (1998) Marital adjustment of older adult couples with breast cancer, prostate cancer, and couples without cancer. *Dissertation Abstracts International: Section B: the Sciences and Engineering*, **59**, 3102.

Index